D1222967

*The Coherence of
Kant's Doctrine of Freedom*

THE Coherence
OF Kant's Doctrine
OF Freedom

BERNARD CARNOIS
Translated by David Booth

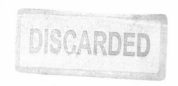

 The University of Chicago Press
Chicago and London

BERNARD CARNOIS was born and educated in France and is
professor of philosophy at the University of Montreal.

Originally published as *La cohérence de la doctrine Kantienne de
la liberté* by Editions du Seuil, © 1973.

The University of Chicago Press, Chicago 60637
The University of Chicago Press, Ltd., London

© 1987 by The University of Chicago
All rights reserved. Published 1987
Printed in the United States of America

96 95 94 93 92 91 90 89 88 87   5 4 3 2 1

Library of Congress Cataloging-in-Publication Data

Carnois, Bernard, 1935–
    The coherence of Kant's doctrine of freedom.

    Translation of: La cohérence de la doctrine
kantienne de la liberté.
        Bibliography: p.
        Includes index.
        1. Kant, Immanuel, 1724–1804—Contributions in free
will and determinism.   2. Free will and determinism.
    I. Title.
B2799.F8C3713   1987   123'.5'0924   86-15935
ISBN 0-226-09394-8

À Monsieur le Professeur

Paul Ricoeur

The concept of freedom, in so far as its reality is established as an apodictic law of practical reason, is the *keystone* of the whole architecture of the system of pure reason and even of speculative reason.

—Kant, *Critique of Practical Reason*

Contents

Acknowledgments

Permit me here to express my gratitude to, and admiration for, Paul Ricoeur, who kindly guided the present work, and who never withheld his advice, his objections, and his encouragement. I would also acknowledge the friendly and enlightening support afforded me throughout the course of my research by Dina Dreyfus and Henri Birault. Thanks are also due to Gilles Deleuze, Martial Gueroult, and Louis Guillermit, who initiated me into the study of transcendental philosophy.

Finally, I would like to acknowledge two organizations which facilitated the editing and contributed to the publication of my work. This book was published with the help of a subsidy granted by the Conseil canadien de recherches sur les humanités from funds furnished by the Conseil des arts du Canada.

Introduction

The idea of freedom occupies a privileged place in Kant's philosophy. We read in the *Critique of Practical Reason* that "it is, properly speaking, only the concept of freedom, among all the ideas of pure speculative reason, which brings [knowledge] such a great extension in the field of the supersensuous."[1] It is a concept deeply connected with our being, and it is precisely because of this connection that we must inquire into its richness. "Only the concept of freedom enables us to find the unconditioned for the conditioned and the intelligible for the sensuous without going outside ourselves."[2] It opens up to us our means of access to the supersensible. Yet all the knowledge which it makes available to us belongs to the practical order. Above all, the concept of freedom concerns action, and especially moral action. "The concept of freedom . . . is the key to the most sublime practical principles for critical moralists."[3] Thus, the concept appears to be fundamental in a twofold sense: it is one of the "foundation stones [*Grundsteine*] of morals and religion";[4] and it "is the keystone [*Schlussstein*] of the whole architecture of the system of pure reason and even of speculative reason."[5]

Yet while this idea of freedom assures the unity and cohesion of the critical system, it presents itself under such disparate aspects that it seems we must admit that Kant's philosophy includes several concepts of freedom, not just a single one. Delbos puts the matter plainly: "Is there only one idea of freedom throughout the 'critical period'? If one takes account of all the texts, it is very difficult to reconstruct it with perfect coherence. Not only do Kant's many works disagree about attributing a single meaning and role to it, that disagreement seems to appear in each of the works taken separately."[6] We are dealing with an absolutely fundamental problem here, since it is precisely on the idea of freedom that the entire critical edifice is constructed. To doubt the coherence of this idea, therefore, is at the same time to doubt the unity and cohesion of Kant's system.

Is Kant's idea of freedom coherent? This is the question we propose to answer. The answer will be affirmative if we succeed in showing that the different concepts of freedom do not contradict one another but are so closely related that their mere multiplicity in no way threatens the unity and harmony of Kant's theory. In his book *La Philosophie pratique de Kant,* Delbos provides a list of the main questions raised by the relations among these different concepts. In large part this list furnishes a program for our reflection.

What is the notion of freedom essential to the *Critique of Pure Reason?* Is it a cosmological freedom, conceived as an idea of reason, and independent of experience? Or is it a practical freedom, known directly through experience? Which of these two types of freedom is related to that freedom which is identical to the autonomous will, and which is required for *the establishment of the metaphysics of morals?* And what is the relation of intelligible freedom (which, according to *Religion within the Limits of Reason Alone,* having already produced evil, converts itself to good) to the autonomous will which, by definition, cannot remove itself from the moral legislation it imposes—or, on the other hand, to the intelligible freedom of the *Critique of Pure Reason,* which is above all possible change, and hence above every possible conversion? What significance does it have that in the *Critique of Practical Reason* freedom is first deduced as a principle but then admitted as a postulate? It is hardly astonishing, under the circumstances, that Kant's theory has been judged obscure and contradictory.[7]

What method is appropriate to the attempt to resolve these problems? Without doubt, the principal task which falls to us consists in distinguishing the different concepts of freedom, illuminating the natural articulation of each one, and determining the relations among them, so that finally we can grasp the entirety in a synoptic vision. Does this mean that it would be a mistake to consider Kant's system first as a definitive whole, and pass over the constantly evolving movement of his thought? Not at all. Since it is true that the genesis of a concept, and the way in which it is introduced in a doctrine, tells us a great deal about the nature of that concept, neglecting the overall structure of the system would deprive us of a perfectly sound aid in acquiring knowledge of the system. Thus we will trace the evolution of Kant's thought; we will fix the circumstances under which the many concepts of freedom appear in his system; and we will establish their civil status, so to speak, by taking note of their date of birth and their mother country. Certainly if such a method were pursued too rigidly, there would be a great risk that it would become an obstacle in the pursuit of our goal. In the first place, it often happens that a text clarifies and, as it were, completes an earlier text, even when there are sufficiently important differences between them to require that we preserve them in the proper historical contexts; in cases of this sort a detour through the later text is plainly justified. Moreover, our method runs the risk of concealing or even evading the very problem we propose to clarify and resolve, for it is all too easy to pretend that an idea is neither coherent nor incoherent simply by appealing to the fact that it is constantly evolving and continually transforming itself. Indeed it is true that the addition of new elements can upset the harmony of a system momentarily. But it is the mark of a vital and fecund doctrine that it is always seeking out its own equilibrium. We can even say that the coherence of an idea manifests itself in large part precisely through its striving toward an equilibrium which is always threatened. In tracing the evolution of Kant's idea of freedom, therefore, we will be careful to determine at each step of the way which elements are definitively integrated into the system. These will constitute a kind of constantly growing core. Thus, we will only gradually attain an overall view of the system. Yet our analysis as a whole will raise the question of the coherence of the doctrine of freedom by noting each occasion when a new and definite datum comes to be integrated in the core. The advantage of this method is that it allows us to grasp the dynamic of Kant's thought, while at the same time enabling us to acquire, bit by bit, a view of the entirety, so as to judge the coherence of its structure.[8]

I.   *FREEDOM AND NATURE*

I   *Transcendental Freedom*

The cosmological problem of freedom

Our first approach to the origin of the idea of freedom is through the Transcendental Dialectic, for the idea does not arise from a rational psychology, in the context of reflections on the human soul, but instead from a rational cosmology, through a critical examination of questions about the world which seem to admit of contradictory answers.

Thus, in the third antinomy the problem of freedom emerges originally as a cosmological problem. Yet we must understand clearly in what sense this is so, and this requires us to consider the way Kant poses the problem. Is there a conflict between the existence of freedom and the demand for an explanation of the world? Since freedom seems to imply an absolute abrogation of the necessity of the laws of nature—and thereby to make the unity of experience impossible—it would, if admitted, destroy our knowledge of nature. It would cut us loose from the laws of nature and deprive us of that guiding thread of rules which permits us to establish the order and connection of events in the world. Put in these terms, the problem of freedom appears to impose itself from outside a rational cosmology. The supposition of transcendental freedom, in the sense of a particular type of causality through which events in the world could take place, would make every explanation of those same events fragile and uncertain. And this would give rise to the cosmological problem of freedom, namely, the question whether it is possible to resolve the apparent contradiction between freedom and natural necessity.

In fact this problem must be called cosmological in a far more radical and basic sense, for it originates in cosmology itself. Far from imposing itself from outside, it is precisely through cosmology that it arises: cosmology is the source of the transcendental idea of freedom. The question at issue is not that of reconciling a previously

admitted freedom with natural necessity, but of resolving a conflict
which arises within reason itself. While it is true that freedom seems
to make our knowledge of the world uncertain, it must not be forgotten that it is precisely in willing to perfect our knowledge of the
world that reason produces the idea of free causality in the first
place. That is why it would be somewhat inexact to say that the idea
of freedom resembles a cosmological problem. Rather we should say
that the idea of freedom *is* a cosmological problem.

The problem is expressed in the form of an antinomy. The explanation of events in the world according to their causes seems to require both the affirmation and the denial of the existence of freedom. Both thesis and antithesis seem to be proved irrefutably. Yet
each cancels the other, and it is vain to expect either to concede
victory to the other. This "entangles reason in an unresolvable conflict"; at the same time, reason plunges "into the most hopeless
scepticism." [1]

By affirming that there is no freedom, and that everything in the
world occurs according to the laws of nature, the antithesis seeks to
preserve the unity of experience. [2] Let the understanding be prudent!
It is better for it to remain on the firm ground of experience, "the
land of truth [*das Land der Wahrheit*]," [3] than to venture into the realm
of reason, "the true empire of illusion [*Sitze des Scheins*]." [4] Indeed,
this warning addressed to the understanding is all the more perti-
nent since the temptation to undertake just such an adventure is so
strong. But if it is true that a free causality interposing itself in the
natural connection of events would render the play of appearances
incoherent, or prevent us from distinguishing dream and reality,
then it is doubtless in the interest of the understanding not to sur-
render to "the illusion of freedom [*das Blendwerk von Freiheit*]." [5] If
there were nothing more than this to the problem, then certainly the
antithesis would win the understanding over.

The thesis, on the other hand, makes it clear that it is not so
simple. What must free causality mean? The thesis answers this
question by describing the origin of the transcendental idea of freedom. At the same time, it discloses that such a free causality is admitted only with the understanding's own blessings. The understanding finds itself torn between two apparently contradictory
demands, the first of which concerns its own most basic task. As a
faculty of cognition and rules, the understanding explains events in

the world by their causes. It unifies the manifold of sensible intuition by linking appearances through causal relations, following the principle that "all alterations take place in conformity with the law of the connection of cause and effect."[6] It thus makes ordered experience possible. Achieving this within the realm of causality completes the work of the understanding. But it hardly completes our knowledge of the world. Indeed, the causality of natural laws never provides us with more than an incomplete determination: when one has discovered the cause of an appearance, it must still be admitted that this cause "must have *begun to act,* otherwise no succession between it and the effect could be thought. Otherwise the effect, as well as the causality [*Kausalität*] of the cause, would have always existed."[7] The latter "is itself, therefore, something that has *taken place,* which again presupposes, in accordance with the law of nature, a preceding state and its causality, and this in similar manner a still earlier state, and so on."[8] The understanding vainly traces each state to a preceding one, since it is never granted to us to grasp the series of causes in its entirety. Through the understanding, we would always apprehend only subsequent beginnings, and never a first beginning. Therefore, the understanding offers us only a partial explanation of appearances, rather than a complete one. To be content with such an explanation would violate the law of nature that determines a priori that nothing happens without a sufficiently determined cause. One must therefore admit an unconditioned causality, "an *absolute spontaneity* of the cause, whereby a series of appearances, which proceeds in accordance with laws of nature, begins *of itself.* This is transcendental freedom, without which, even in the [ordinary] course of nature, the series of appearances on the side of the causes can never be complete."[9]

Such is the second demand imposed on the understanding: to permit reason to pursue to the end the work it has undertaken but has not been able to complete. The main task of reason is to investigate the entire, completed unity of cognition. Where the understanding is the power of gathering appearances into a unity by means of rules, reason is the faculty of gathering the rules of the understanding into a unity by means of principles. It realizes this rational unity by producing certain concepts (which Kant calls "transcendental ideas") which express the unconditioned, or the absolute totality of conditions. In this way, reason, in pursuing the explanation

of appearances by their causes, produces the idea of an absolute
spontaneity of causes in order to make it a priori possible for us to
embrace an entire series of conditions. This is not meant to offend
the understanding. On the contrary, the affirmation of transcendental freedom "offers a point of *rest* to the enquiring understanding in
the chain of causes, conducting *it* to an unconditioned causality
which begins to act of itself." [10] But this "point of rest" offered to the
understanding is quite deceptive. Doesn't reason, in willing to perfect the work carried out by the understanding, actually run the risk
of destroying it?

The idea of freedom demanded by the search for a complete explanation of events in the world seems to undermine that very explanation. Such is the cosmological problem which emerges in the
third antinomy. It is worth noting that this problem seems to break
through the limits of the scheme in which it was originally contained. "In Kant's thought," Brunschvicg writes, "the attribution of
freedom to the *first causality,* which in his view lends an interest to
the dogmatic *thesis,* implies a double shift of the cosmological problem: on one hand, a shift into the realm of psychology, and on the
other, a shift into the realm of theology." [11] This is an apt remark if
it is not presented as a reproach to Kant. To say that the problem
undergoes a shift does not necessarily amount to a charge that there
was, in Kant's mind, a confusion of distinct spheres. It only indicates
that the problem first built up on the ground of cosmology extends
also into other spheres, not that it breaks down the framework of
rational cosmology, as Brunschvicg contends. In other words, there
is a partial fusion of certain realms, not a transition from one to
another.

First, the problem extends into the sphere of theology. In order
to account for the reality of the world, a sufficiently determined
cause must be admitted a priori. This is a requirement of reason. In
the same way, the philosophers of antiquity felt themselves compelled to admit a prime mover in order to explain the movement of
the world. Without freedom the world would only be possible: in
order to conceive it as real, we have to assume an original spontaneity from which the whole series of appearances would derive.
"The necessity of a first beginning, due to freedom, of a series of
appearances we have demonstrated only in so far as it is required to
make an *origin of the world* conceivable." [12] Kant is speaking here of an

absolutely first beginning, both in regard to time and in regard to causality. The reference to a prime mover and the appeal to an original spontaneity witness to the close ties linking the third antinomy both to the fourth antinomy and to the ideal of pure reason. Kant himself emphasizes these ties when he says that "reason . . . by means of the *theological* Idea . . . leads to the concept of a cause possessing freedom, and then to that of a Supreme Intelligence."[13] At the same time, the accent in the third antinomy is not placed on the existence of a necessary being, but on its causality, its power of being a first cause, and on the fact that through these it provides a principle for explaining events in the world. Thus the problem remains a cosmological one even when extended.

In the same manner it is correct to affirm that the cosmology does not immediately pass over into the question of human freedom, but that human freedom appears as a more general statement of the cosmological problem. Once one has admitted an absolute spontaneity, as required to make an origin of the world conceivable, "it is now also possible for us to admit [*so ist es uns nunmehr auch erlaubt*] *within the course of the world* different series as capable in their causality of beginning of themselves, and so to attribute to their substances a power of acting from freedom."[14] In responding to the objection that "no absolute first beginning [*absolut erster Anfang*] of a series is possible during the course of the world," Kant states clearly that he is talking about an absolutely first beginning with respect to causality, not with respect to time.[15] When, for example, I arise from my chair, quite freely and without being subject to any necessary determination of natural causes, I initiate a particular series of events. Doubtless this free action, occurring "during the course of the world," *follows on* natural causes, but it does not *derive* from them. The spontaneity of thinking beings may thus appear as a principle for explaining certain events in the world, so it is not surprising that cosmology passes over into the question of human freedom. Moreover, the answer cosmology provides to this question will be of the greatest interest to morals, insofar as the freedom of the thinking self is one of the "foundation stones of morals and religion."[16]

New perspectives appear to us now. The horizon which opens out onto psychology and morals will assume such importance and magnitude in Kant's eyes that the cosmological problem, once the conflict is resolved, will apparently pass to the second rank. Still, we should not be misled: this is the same problem which, in the third antinomy, is at the origin of the question of human freedom. Even when Kant treats moral and voluntary actions more particularly, he does not break the framework of rational cosmology, since the spontaneity of the thinking self appears there, too, as a principle for explaining certain events in the world.

The solution of the antinomy

We encounter here two assertions, neither of which is any less rigorously grounded on account of their dialectical relation. Kant never hesitates to affirm that "the thesis, as well as the antithesis, can be shown by equally clear, evident, and irresistible proofs—for I pledge myself as to the correctness of all these proofs."[17] Thus the problem is posed as sharply as it can be. And the reader, once swept up in Kant's arguments, can hardly fail to appreciate the drama of the question. Nevertheless, Kant is too deeply convinced that our faculties are well constituted not to presume that the source of such a conflict is "a simple misunderstanding,"[18] which will dissolve with the elimination of "the scandal of reason's apparent self-contradiction."[19] The study of the third antinomy enables us to illuminate the nature of this vexatious mistake.

As we approach the critical solution Kant provides to the antinomy, it will be useful to emphasize that the question is not presented as a disjunctive proposition, calling on us to choose between natural necessity and freedom, as if every effect in the world had to result either from nature or from freedom. If the question were in that form, the answer would certainly have been found already and the debate swiftly settled. The Transcendental Dialectic, after all, was preceded by the Analytic, whose results we dare not ignore. Thus it should come as no surprise that Kant thought it worthwhile to remind us that the principle of causality constitutes "a law of the understanding, from which no departure can be permitted [*under any circumstances*], and from which no appearance may be exempted."[20] "That all events in the sensible world stand in thoroughgoing connection in accordance with unchangeable laws of nature is an established principle of the Transcendental Analytic, *and allows of no exception*."[21] The antithesis thus seems to enjoy an undeniable advantage at the outset, since the thing which constitutes its truth and its power, the thing it so sharply and intransigently affirms, is just this principle of causality. It believes it can conclude that there is no freedom. But it remains to be seen if this is a legitimate conclusion. The question which arises—and after Kant it cannot be overstressed—concerns the "possibility of Causality through Freedom, in Harmony with the Universal Law of Natural Necessity." [22] "The question, therefore, can only be whether freedom is completely excluded by this inviolable rule, or whether an effect, notwithstanding its being thus determined in accordance with nature, may not at the same time be grounded in freedom." [23] "The only question here is this:—Admitting that in the whole series of events there is nothing but natural necessity, is it not possible to regard one and the same event as being in one aspect merely an effect of nature and in another aspect an effect due to freedom; or is there between these two kinds of causality a direct contradiction?" [24]

Once the problem is formulated this way, the path to a critical solution of the antinomy is clear. It cannot be disputed that appearances are bound together according to the universal law of natural causality. As a result, it is impossible to find freedom among them. Every effort to reconcile nature and freedom is hopeless so long as one admits, as common opinion is inclined to, that appearances have absolute reality. If there are only appearances, or in other terms, "if appearances are things in themselves," then "freedom cannot be upheld." [25] The principle of causality must be extended to all things, considered as efficient causes. But this common opinion, although utterly devastating for freedom, had already been set aside in the Transcendental Aesthetic, where it was proved that all objects of experience are mere appearances, or simple representations "which . . . have no independent existence outside our thoughts." [26]

Appearances do not make up the whole of reality. Moreover, as mere appearances they must have a ground (*Grund*) which is not itself an appearance, but rather a transcendental object which determines them as representations. "We may entitle the purely intelligible cause of appearances in general the transcendental object" [27]—"the transcendental object lying at the basis of appearances." [28] Appearances are capable of having intelligible causes because of the essentially synthetic character of the category of causality, for causality does not require the homogeneity of the condition and the thing conditioned in their synthesis: cause and effect need not be "of the same type [*gleichartig*]." [29] To measure the significance of this claim, we should consider the "essential distinction"[30] between the mathematical and the dynamical which cuts across the entire critique. We encounter it first at the level of the categories and principles, and then rediscover it in the antithetical, where it proves particularly valuable to reason in the solution of antinomies.[31] The mathematical categories (those of quantity and quality) relate to objects of intuition and simply concern the unity of the synthesis in the representation of these objects. The dynamical categories (those of causality and necessity) concern the existence of objects of intuition and the unity of the synthesis in the representation of the existence of these objects. But the synthesis is different in each case: the mathematical categories always comprise a synthesis of the *homogeneous* (*Gleichartigen*), while the dynamical categories permit instead a synthesis of the *heterogeneous* (*Ungleichartigen*).[32] This explains why it would be impossible to find the unconditioned in the mathematical antinomies, for the mathematical connection of series of appearances precludes our introducing any other than a sensible condition, that is, a condition which is itself part of a series. By contrast, "in the dynamical series of sensible conditions, a heterogeneous condition, not itself a part of the series, but *purely intelligible,* and as such *outside the series,* can be allowed. In this way reason obtains satisfaction and the unconditioned is set prior to the appearances while yet the invariably conditioned character of the appearances is not obscured, nor their series cut short, in violation of the principles prescribed by the understanding."[33] It follows that nothing precludes our attributing to the transcendental object, "besides [*ausser*] the quality in terms of which it appears, a *causality* [*auch eine Kausalität*] which is not appearance, although its effect is to be met with in appearance."[34] Such an intelligible cause (*intelligible Ursache*), in the same way as its unconditioned causality (*Kausalität*), is therefore *outside* the series, while its effects occur *within* the series of empirical conditions.

In this manner we can envision a double reading of each event. On one hand, it is permissible, according to the demands of scientific understanding, to link each event to the preceding appearances which determine it and locate it in the flow of physical necessity. On the other hand, it would be legitimate to conceive it as the effect of an intelligible cause, without thereby claiming to know this supersensible cause or the relation which connects it to its sensible effect. "Thus the effect may be regarded as free in respect of its intelligible cause, and at the same time in respect of appearances as resulting from them according to the necessity of nature."[35] Correlatively, the causality of a being could be envisioned according to two points of view: as *intelligible* in respect to its action considered as the action of a thing in itself; and as *sensible* in respect to the effects of this action considered as appearances in the sensible world.

Here then are the two principles which make possible a resolution of the third antinomy: the distinction between things-in-themselves and appearances; and the possibility of thinking a causal relation between things-in-themselves and appearances, in spite of the unavoidable heterogeneity of the condition and the thing conditioned.[36] The first principle offers the key to the four antinomies. The second, for its part, applies only to the dynamical antinomies, but for these it empowers a highly original solution. Since the category of causality permits a synthesis of the heterogeneous, an altogether new perspective opens up to us, and the "suit" in which reason is engaged "may be settled to the satisfaction of both parties."[37] The antinomy is in no way avoided in favor of any negative solution, suppressing either of the two opposed terms, nor again in favor of any conciliatory solution, identifying either of the terms with the other. The two terms are preserved in their own spheres, and they remain distinct.

To the question whether it is possible to harmonize free causality and natural causality, Kant replies that in the third antinomy "the falsehood of the presupposition consists in representing as contradictory what is compatible."[38] Here we are in the presence of a *dialectical opening*. The two affirmations "may *both* alike be *true* [*wahr sein können*],"[39] provided that we have correctly understood them. The antithesis rightly insists that appearances are strictly linked according to natural causality. But properly speaking, this law of the understanding is valid only in the world of appearances, and not for things-in-themselves. For its part, the thesis rightly addresses reason's demand that something unconditioned be placed at the beginning of all appearances. But it commits the error of placing this unconditioned something in the series of appearances, rather than outside it on the noumenal plane. Once modified, thesis and antithesis come into agreement: the antithesis is true, but the thesis *could* be true also. If we notice here a difference in the degree of assent granted to each, we must take it only as a reflection of the finitude of our intellect; it is capable of thinking (*denken*) things-in-themselves, but not of knowing (*erkennen*) them. We will return to this point, but for now it is most important to maintain that, thanks to such a "settlement," both understanding and reason may be satisfied. The understanding will never permit an empirically unconditioned condition among the appearances; nevertheless, one can conceive an empirically unconditioned condition which would be intelligible, and which as a result would not belong to the series of appearances.[40] Thus, this nontemporal causality does not interrupt the chain of phenomenal causes but, being unconditioned, it provides us with an explanation of the entire series, or of a particular series of events without thereby rendering the unity of experience impossible. The work of the understanding is thus protected while being accomplished by reason in a particular manner which we will have to specify.

One result of the solution of the third antinomy is that freedom can be attributed only to beings which are not mere appearances but things-in-themselves. Such a being would have a purely intelligible power permitting it to determine its action, not under empirical influence, but solely under principles of the understanding. Nothing prevents us from supposing the existence of such beings. But the supposition would remain a pure fiction if we were not able to verify it thanks to the knowledge we have of ourselves.

In lifeless, or merely animal, nature we find no ground for thinking that any faculty is conditioned otherwise than in a merely sensible manner. Man, however, who knows all the rest of nature solely through the senses, knows himself also through pure apperception; and this, indeed, in acts and inner determinations which he cannot regard as impressions of the senses. He is thus to himself, on the one hand phenomenon, and on the other hand, in respect of certain faculties the action of which cannot be ascribed to the receptivity of sensibility, a purely intelligible object.[41]

Kant does not specify what this nonempirical apperception consists in. Doubtless we must distinguish it from the pure, original apperception "which produces the representation *I think*,"[42] and which accompanies every empirical perception. The apperception in question here permits man to know himself as a noumenon. What does this mean? In order not to misrepresent the meaning of the text, we must insist that the knowledge of a noumenon, whatever it might be, escapes the grasp of our understanding. Such knowledge would only be possible for an "understanding which should know its object, not discursively through categories, but intuitively in a non-sensible intuition."[43] All intellectual intuition is precluded for us. The understanding must impose limits on itself and at the same time limit sensation in calling things-in-themselves noumena. It is curious that this same understanding, which cannot lay claim to any knowledge of noumena, nevertheless rightly authorizes man to consider himself as a noumenon.[44] Man "is to himself an intelligible object."[45] This does not mean that he knows *what* he, as noumenal, is; but he knows *that* he is a noumenon. Indeed, man has the privilege of considering himself a noumenon, but he "may not presume to know even himself as he really is."[46] Put another way, I can without contradiction affirm that certain aspects of myself are unknowable by me, but not that I can know these unknowable aspects.[47]

A human being is for himself both a sensible and a supersensible being, both phenomenon and noumenon. The faculties which lift him above the merely sensible are the understanding and reason— reason "in particular," Kant specifies.[48] The latter is objectively *determinable,* which means that it can be determined by the objective principles which are the pure ideas. Considering effects in the sensible world, these principles are taken as *determinative.* This is how, mediated through ideas, the causality of reason operates: it is the free causality of an objectively determinable and determinative faculty. But in speaking of freedom we speak of the capability of spontaneously beginning a series of events. Indeed it is a question of a nontemporal causality. "For the relation of the action to objective grounds of reason is not a time-relation; in this case that which determines the causality does not precede in time the action, because such determining grounds represent, not a reference to objects of sense, e.g., to causes in the appearances, but to determining causes as things in themselves, which do not stand under conditions of time."[49] Moreover, this rational causality is perfectly reconcilable with natural causality, as it implies no diminution of the necessity of natural laws. We can envision two cases in which a rational subject acts, or does not act, by virtue of rational principles. In the first case, "reason is the cause of these laws of nature";[50] thus, the effect is still determined according to unchanging laws. In the second case, "the effects follow according to mere natural laws of sensibility";[51] here reason remains free, but its influence is, in a manner of speaking, suspended. Hence, there is no contradiction whatsoever in attribut-

ing both nature and freedom to one and the same being considered
from two different perspectives, since in these two cases reason remains free, yet still "the law of nature remains."[52]

The solution to the third antinomy thus applies to reasonable beings in particular. But to be quite precise, it is not that such an "application"[53] would be absolutely necessary, as if it were crucial to
confirm the solution to the cosmological problem by basing it on
"properties which we *meet* in the actual world."[54] It is only a question here of giving "an *example* to make the thing intelligible."[55] Yet it
is on this basis that the cosmological problem opens up into the
realms of psychology and morals. The expression Kant uses for this
subject is significant. Certain "properties which we meet in the actual world," particularly in ourselves, disclose the conflict of freedom and necessity to us. In this sense we can say that the antinomy
presents to us a *lived antinomy*. It seems reason's causality crops up at
the level of consciousness. Our experience attests to it; and therein
our practical freedom is revealed to us. Practical freedom, however,
far from providing yet another solution to the conflict, is itself based
on the transcendental idea of freedom. We should not, therefore,
pose as a solution to the conflict something which, as an example,
merely illustrates that solution. Likewise we can consider intelligible
character as one application of the transcendental idea of freedom to
human will. These two concepts of practical freedom and intelligible
character suggest two directions toward which we will be able to
orient ourselves once the answer to the cosmological question has
been elucidated. For now, it will be enough to have indicated the
close connection between them and cosmological freedom.

Apparently we are not to identify intelligible causality and free
causality absolutely. The concept of freedom is in effect a relational
one. It does not present itself in the intelligible as such, but rather in
a certain relation: "The Idea of freedom occurs only in the relation
of the intellectual as cause, to the appearance, as effect."[56] In other
words, an intelligible cause can only be considered free to the extent
that it determines a cause to produce a sensible effect. As a result,
our concept of freedom does not suit "purely rational beings, for
instance, . . . God, so far as his action is immanent."[57] This idea
qualifies both the *relation* of causality and the *terms* of that relation.
But there must be a relation through which the terms—the cause
and the effect—could receive this qualification. If the effect itself

"may be regarded as free," it is only "*in respect of* its intelligible cause." [58] As for the cause which is part of a series of conditions, or which at least is not altogether outside the series, it can be called free *in respect of* its causality, since "only its *causality* was thought as intelligible." [59] Intelligible causality, or causality outside the sensible, is free to the extent that it produces an appearance. God, who is a "purely rational being," [60] "*ens extramundum,*" [61] cannot be called free *insofar as* his action is immanent and remains, as it were, enclosed within the intelligible with no relation to the sensible. The idea of freedom only emerges in the relation between an intelligible causality and its effect in the sensible world. The definition of freedom as a "faculty of starting an event spontaneously" [62] expresses this perfectly. As Delbos accurately observes: "The idea of a first beginning is of value neither in the world of things-in-themselves (where nothing begins), nor in the world of appearances (where nothing is first) exclusively. Its value is to signify the causality of the first with respect to the second." [63]

The concept of transcendental freedom

Following the exposition of the antinomy and the solution provided by the critical philosophy, we are in a position to specify the status of the transcendental idea of freedom. In depicting how the idea arises, the thesis has already provided us with valuable information in this regard, but it threatens to lead us into error if we do not proceed carefully. The following analysis aims to show how Kant wards off this threat and clears up the illusion which proceeds from reason's misunderstanding with itself. [64]

Human reason is ambitious: it strives to furnish a complete explanation of appearances and seeks to attain the unconditioned. [65] There is nothing illegitimate in this ambition in itself: indeed, it is "by necessity and by right," as Kant says, that reason demands the unconditioned for everything that is conditioned, in order thus to complete the series of conditions. [66] Under the circumstances, however, reason cannot rely on the understanding to satisfy this ambition, since the understanding cannot ascend from condition to condition, nor can it ever attain an unconditioned causality, nor can it ever obtain the absolute totality of conditions. [67] Yet reason needs a causality determined in itself for every series of conditions. That is why "reason creates for itself the idea of a spontaneity which can begin to act of itself, without requiring to be determined to action by an antecedent cause in accordance with the law of causality."[68] This is the origin of the transcendental idea of freedom. Like all rational concepts, the idea derives subjectively from the *nature* of reason.

But if the concept of freedom answers to a demand of speculative reason which is both legitimate and unavoidable, does that not authorize us to affirm that the concept represents an undeniable *speculative* interest?[69] Granted, there is in the Canon of Pure Reason a text which seems, if not to forbid, at least to undermine such an interpretation. Evidently Kant affirms that, in the question of freedom, "the merely speculative interest of reason is very small,"[70] given that the discoveries one might make in this area would be of no use in the study of nature. But clearly this text does not present his last word on the matter. In the Transcendental Dialectic, Kant does not fail to emphasize the advantages which the theses in the Antinomies present in the domain of knowledge:

The propositions of the antithesis are of such a kind that they render the completion of the edifice of knowledge quite impossible. They maintain that there is always to be found beyond every state of the world a more ancient state, in every part yet other parts similarly divisible, prior to every event still another event which itself again is likewise generated, and that in existence in general everything is conditioned, an unconditioned and first existence being nowhere discernible. Since, therefore, the antithesis thus refuses to admit as first or as a beginning anything that could serve as a foundation for building, a complete edifice of knowledge is, on such assumptions, altogether impossible. Thus the architectonic interest of reason—the demand not for empirical but for pure *a priori* unity of reason—forms a natural recommendation for the assertions of the thesis.[71]

Beyond a merely practical interest, therefore, "reason has a *speculative interest* on the side of the thesis. When the transcendental ideas are postulated and employed in the manner prescribed by the thesis, the entire chain of conditions and the derivation of the conditioned can be grasped completely a priori. For we then start from the unconditioned."[72] Later, a second *Critique* will reaffirm that reason in its theoretical employment requires the concept of freedom. And it does not hesitate to use an expression which can be found already in the thesis: the concept of freedom is needed by speculative reason.[73] Here we encounter again what we have seen before—namely, freedom's "indispensability . . . in the complete use of speculative reason."[74]

The idea of freedom is a natural and necessary concept for reason: it is impossible for reason *not* to conceive it. Yet at the same time the idea exposes reason to a "*natural* and inevitable *illusion.*"[75] Thus, in a quite general way, the transcendental ideas can be misleading in virtue of the powerful tendency which impels us to take them for concepts of real things, and so to presume to gain access through their mediation to a knowledge of realities situated beyond the limits of possible experience. It is important to bear in mind here that knowledge requires two elements: intuitions and concepts. For an object to be known, the concept, by which the object is thought, must be completed by the intuition, which provides us with the contents of knowledge. Apart from intuition, the concept remains empty. Since, on the other side, the understanding is always discursive, and never intuitive, all intellectual intuition is impossible for us. Our nature is so constituted that intuition can never be anything but sensible. As a result, our knowledge is limited to the domain of experience. Reason, however, is hardly willing to concede these evident restrictions. Forgetting its finitude, it cherishes the pretension of knowing supersensible realities. Although the idea of freedom is "a necessary concept of reason to which no corresponding object can be given in sense-experience,"[76] reason persists in "assuming that there is an actual object corresponding to the idea."[77] And although the idea is a "transcendent concept,"[78] which surpasses the limits of all experience, reason persists in attributing objective reality to it,[79] for "possible experience is that which can alone give reality to our concepts; in its absence a concept is a mere idea, without truth, that is, without relation to any object."[80]

To forget that the idea of freedom is *only* an idea is to succumb to the illusion Kant names "the illusion of freedom."[81] In order to satisfy its need—its demand—for the unconditioned, reason claims to ascertain the existence of a free causality by appealing to the mere idea of freedom, as if the need could be a proof of the reality which fulfills it. Plainly this is an illegitimate claim, for "freedom is *only* an *idea* of reason whose objective reality in itself is doubtful."[82] The concept of freedom is a "transcendent concept,"[83] and so "indemonstrable."[84] No intuition corresponds to it. Hence freedom, considered "as a property of a being to which I attribute effects in the sensible world, is therefore unknowable in any such fashion. For I should then have to know such a being as determined in its existence, and yet as not determined in time—which is impossible, since I cannot support my concept by any intuition." [85]

Here reason is dislodged from that illusory repose in which it was sustained by the claim to know freedom. This repose, let us not forget, was also enjoyed by the understanding. "The illusion of freedom . . . offers a point of rest to the enquiring understanding in the chain of causes, conducting it to an unconditioned causality which begins to act of itself." [86] This is to say that the understanding does not find satisfaction only in the antithesis. This point deserves to be emphasized. Evidently we are in a position to affirm that the antinomy of freedom and natural necessity consists less in an opposition between reason and the understanding than in a conflict which divides reason against itself, and which affects the understanding, above and beyond reason. The understanding is less in conflict with reason than "seduced" by it: "the transcendental Ideas . . . seduce the understanding by an unavoidable illusion to a transcendent use." [87] Once invited by reason to venture out of the domain of sensible experience ("forced out of its sphere" [88]), the errant understanding begins to stray (schwärmen), and allows itself to be led into a desire to taste of the tree of supersensible knowledge—a knowledge which is both impossible and illegitimate for ordinary people (nous autres hommes).

If Kant insists on specifying that the Transcendental Dialectic, in resolving the antinomy, does not claim "to establish the reality of freedom as one of the faculties which contain the cause of the appearances of our sensible world," [89] it is to put us once more on guard against the illusion of freedom. For it is an illusion so "prized and cherished" [90] that it could well turn the results of the dialectic to its own use and attempt by specious arguments to find a firmer foundation for itself. After all, can we not deduce from the fact that freedom and natural necessity are not contradictory the fact that freedom is real? Yet between these two affirmations there extends the enormous distance which separates the logical possibility of a concept from the reality of its object. And Kant always avoids traversing that distance.

If we cannot know freedom, then, can we at least think it? We know that in order to think an object it is not necessary for it to be given us in an intuition: the mere concept suffices, so long as it is not self-contradictory. "I can *think* whatever I please, provided only that I do not contradict myself, that is, provided my concept is a possible thought."[91] But it was precisely the *logical possibility* of the concept of freedom which was put in doubt by the third antinomy. The contradiction which seemed to exist between freedom and the mechanism of nature turned out to be merely apparent, however. Indeed, we can attribute freedom and nature to a single being, considered according to different relations. In this way a conflict which menaced reason in its very essence, and plunged it into an abyss of skepticism, was dissolved. It was important to prove that reason in its demand for the unconditioned was not constrained to think the unthinkable, or to conceive the inconceivable, in order to satisfy its need[92]—a prudent precaution, which saves us from folly by permitting us to think.[93] Thus, "though I cannot *know,* I can yet *think* freedom; that is to say, the representation of it is at least not self-contradictory."[94]

It remains no less true, however, that this concept, while non-contradictory, may yet be empty. Assuredly, its object may be distinguished from the *nihil negativum,*[95] insofar as it acquires a sort of existence in thought. The emptiness of a concept includes a positive element, since the concept is now disposed to receive the data which may come to fill it. But at the level of the Transcendental Dialectic, the thought of freedom remains empty—that is, without content. It receives no determination whatsoever, so that we can not know if the concept is related to a real object and if, as a result, it signifies anything.[96] The *real or transcendental possibility* of freedom is not proved, since the objective value of its concept remains uncertain; and we have no right to conclude the real possibility of its object from the logical possibility of a concept. "For the possibility of the concept of a thing (that the concept does not contradict itself) is not sufficient for admitting the possibility of the thing itself (the objective reality of the concept)."[97]

What we have just said can clarify certain passages which may cause confusion, since when Kant talks about the possibility of freedom, he does not always specify whether it is a matter of logical possibility or real possibility. Thus, for instance, he maintains that speculative reason "had to *assume* [*anzunehmen*] at least the [logical] possibility of freedom,"[98] since "the idea of freedom as a faculty of absolute spontaneity was not just a desideratum but, as far as its [logical] possibility was concerned, an analytical principle of pure speculation," [99] despite the fact that freedom is a concept "the [real] possibility of which it could not otherwise venture to affirm." [100] It is permissible for us to *conceive* (*denken*) freedom, but not to *assume* (*anzunehmen*) it; for freedom is a supersensible object, and "to assume the possibility of a supersensible Being determined according to certain concepts would be a completely groundless supposition." [101] The confrontation and *rapprochement* between these apparently contradictory texts allows us to clarify these terms and fix their meaning more precisely.

The concept of freedom thus fits Kant's definition of a "problematic concept" well: it "cannot be in any way known, while yet [it] contains no contradiction." [102] Certainly it is not unthinkable that an object might be related to such an idea. All we know is that the object could not be known by any mode supplied by sensibility. In this sense it is well to affirm that speculative philosophy "could give merely a negative concept of freedom." [103] Freedom is not phenomenal—it is not situated in time, nor can it be grasped by sensible intuition. But this negative employment of the concept of freedom does not admit of a positive counterpart, for the concept remains empty. No sensible object will ever fill this emptiness (in this sense the concept of freedom is a limiting concept). And while it is not unthinkable that it might be filled by a supersensible object, the problem as such remains itself and proves insoluble in the theoretical domain (in this sense the concept of freedom is a problematic concept). [104] Freedom is a supersensible object which reason "could think." [105] Such a thought is a problematical judgment—that is, it is a judgment for which both the affirmation and the denial are admissible merely as possible (or arbitrary). [106] Indeed, the concept of freedom, as a problematic concept, "is the representation of a thing of which we can neither say that it is possible nor that it is impossible." [107] The critical operation has at least established that, if it is not possible to prove freedom, neither is it possible to deny it:

> Whenever I hear that a writer of real ability has demonstrated away the
> freedom of the human will, the hope of a future life, and the existence of
> God, I am eager to read the book, for I expect him by his talents to
> increase my insight into these matters. Already, before having opened it, I
> am perfectly certain that he has not justified any one of his specific claims;
> not because I believe that I am in possession of conclusive proofs of these
> important propositions, but because the transcendental critique, which

has disclosed to me all the resources of our pure reason, has completely convinced me that, as reason is incompetent to arrive at affirmative assertions in this field, it is equally unable, indeed even less able, to establish any negative conclusion in regard to these questions.[108]

In this context it seems legitimate to apply to freedom the expression "rational belief,"[109] which Kant employs to characterize the requirement of reason in its theoretical use. Nevertheless, the reservations which must condition our acceptance of such an expression are already familiar to us. Under pain of introducing "contraband"[110] into the field of speculative knowledge, it is crucial to specify that the hypothesis of freedom is incapable of replacing an objective principle of explanation for real appearances. How can something which is inexplicable and problematic fill such a function? "A *transcendental hypothesis,* in which a mere idea of reason is used in explanation of natural existences, would really be no explanation; so to proceed would be to explain something, which in terms of known empirical principles we do not understand sufficiently, by something which we do not understand at all."[111] The satisfaction and "point of rest" which reason would know thereby would be purely illusory. By what right can reason claim to have accomplished its task, which is the perfection of knowledge, if whenever natural explanation becomes difficult it resorts to "a transcendental ground of explanation which relieves us from further investigation"?[112] Through this empty claim reason attempts both to conceal and to justify its own indolence, which leads it to "dream," or to "play with thoughts," instead of thinking.[113] But the reason which judges reason is scarcely fooled. It denounces this playful and dreamlike activity, which inevitably fascinates the indolent reason, by disclosing what reason is and ought to be, that is, a *reason in need* (*raison besogneuse*), which can satisfy its need only in and through labor.[114]

In the supersensible sphere, the legitimate activity of speculative reason necessarily assumes a negative aspect, for all knowledge of the supersensible is prohibited. And it falls to reason to insure that this prohibition is never transgressed. Without doubt it is necessary to proscribe every transcendent employment of the ideas of reason, which aspires to extend our knowledge beyond the field of experience by claiming to establish, for example, the existence of the soul, of freedom, and of God. But it is crucial nevertheless to dispose of the opposite assertions, which are every bit as illegitimate. To do this, reason quite correctly uses its own ideas, in the form of hypotheses, not so much to promote them as opinions, as to refute opposed opinions. "Hypotheses are therefore, in the domain of pure reason, permissible only as weapons of war, and only for the purpose of defending a right, not in order to establish it."[115] From this perspective it is clear that the hypothesis of freedom is not at all a thesis which might feign a certain degree of probability, but a pure problematic judgment intended to destroy the arguments of those who maintain that one can establish that there is no freedom. It is employed to neutralize the opponent. In reason's speculative employment, "the hypotheses . . . are merely *problematic* judgments, which at least cannot be refuted, although they do not indeed allow of any proof."[116]

Considering only the polemical employment of reason, it would evidently be difficult to sustain Kant's claim that all knowledge is achieved within the limits of reason. If reason is to play a positive role in knowledge, it must necessarily be able to pursue its activity in the field of experience. Transcendental concepts must lend themselves to an immanent use.[117] While the transcendent use of rational concepts would transform the supersensible sphere into a veritable "home of illusion" where reason thinks it can venture, their immanent use restores reason to the "land of truth" where it completes the task assigned to it, in order thus to be able to reap "the fruits that spring from the cultivation of *its own proper domain,* namely, that of experience."[118] In this "territory of pure understanding,"[119] however, reason does not claim to substitute itself for the understanding in order to accomplish the work of knowledge by itself. It only stipulates the rules which serve as a canon for the understanding. "The understanding does not [by this canon] obtain more knowledge of any object than it would have by means of its own concepts, but for the acquiring of such knowledge it receives better and more extensive guidance."[120] The ideas of reason make possible no objective knowledge, whether this be within or outside of the domain of experience; they serve merely as rules for the understanding, indicating the path it should follow in the domain of experience and stimulating it to extend its use in this direction. In this sense the idea of freedom has no constitutive employment, but, like the other ideas, "an excellent, and indeed indispensably necessary, regulative employment."[121] It is not at all an objective principle, but a maxim of speculative reason.[122] In this regard it assumes a double task. On one hand, it leads the understanding to pursue the inquiry into the conditions of natural appearances, "an enquiry which is to be regarded as never allowing of completion, just *as if* the series of appearances were in itself endless, without any first or supreme member."[123] Thus it preserves us from the error which would incline us to consider the investigation of nature, and especially the explanation of the events of this world, as completed. But on the other hand, it enables us to conceive an unconditioned causality apart from the sensible, which by itself is capable of beginning a series of appearances such that the series "can therefore be regarded *as if* it had an absolute beginning, through an intelligible cause."[124] The "as if [*als ob*]" emphasizes the problematic character of the concept of freedom and warns us against every dogmatic assertion. More fundamentally, it indicates that the "industrious" reason, in contrast to the "indolent" reason, continues to turn to the unconditioned (which it bears as an inward demand), but without claiming to attain it.[125]

Rational concepts, far from being "superfluous and void,"[126] have "their own good and appropriate vocation."[127] In illuminating the regulative use of the ideas of reason, Kant provides the only form of a transcendental deduction possible for such concepts.[128] The ideas of reason are justified by their legitimate, immanent employment; they ought to have some "objective validity, no matter how indeterminate that validity may be."[129] They have an object in some sense, but that object is situated beyond experience and remains problematic. We proceed *as if* an object corresponded to the idea—a purely "heuristic fiction"[130] with the aim of showing us not "how an object is constituted, but how, under its guidance, we should *seek* to determine the constitution and connection of the objects of experience."[131] The idea of freedom, like all the ideas of reason, is invested with a heuristic validity. It possesses a relative objective reality.[132]

As we have already seen from the enunciation of the thesis in the Antinomies, the transcendental idea of freedom presents a practical interest. The idea can serve as a regulative idea, in relation to the evaluation of morality in reasonable beings, by permitting us to conceive in such beings the existence of a ground which justifies judgments of imputability. This is the aspect we must study now, as we proceed to the analysis of the concepts of practical freedom and intelligible character.

2   *Practical Freedom*

Practical freedom is defined essentially by the rationality of willing. The human will is an *arbitrium sensitivum*—that is, a sensuous will—insofar as it is affected by sensuous motives. But these motives never render its action necessary. Thus it is not an *arbitrium brutum* but an *arbitrium liberum*. Sensuous motives affect the human will but do not determine it; and the independence from "coercion through sensuous impulses" defines practical freedom.[1] This is a negative definition, however, and as such it expresses the essence of freedom less well than another definition (which nonetheless follows from it): "A will which can be determined independently of sensuous impulses, and therefore through motives which are represented only by reason, is entitled *free will* (*arbitrium liberum*), and everything which is bound up with this will, whether as ground or as consequence, is entitled *practical*."[2]

Thus, we have a power of determining ourselves apart from the coercion of sensuous impulses. This power is reason. A will determined by reason is free. Everything which is possible through freedom is entitled "practical." Experience testifies to this sort of freedom. We can verify in ourselves that our will, through the representation of what is useful and what is detrimental, has the ability to rise above sensible impressions. "These considerations, as to what is desirable in respect of our whole state, that is, as to what is good and useful, are based on reason."[3] Thanks to this ability, man—unlike the animals—is not tied to the present: he can make judgments in terms of the future. Moreover, rather than submit to a tyranny of *partial* (*partielle*) impressions or, in this sense, a prejudiced (*partiales*) determination, the human being has the power to inquire specifically about what seems desirable in relation to the *totality* of his being. This power of reason which characterizes practical freedom is demonstrated by experience, for I grasp it in myself immediately, by a psychological apprehension, whenever my will conflicts with my sensibility and imposes its veto on the impressions of the senses. From this rational consideration of the good and the useful are born those imperative prescriptions which constitute the objective laws of freedom.[4]

The objective laws of freedom express *what ought to happen,* whereas natural laws pertain only to *what happens.* By 1770, Kant had already presented this classical distinction between what is and what ought to be by opposing the theoretical domain to the practical domain. "We regard a thing theoretically so far as we attend only to what pertains to *existence;* but practically if we consider what, through freedom, *ought* to be in it."[5] Experience discloses to us that a human being has the power to determine itself by reason, independently of sensuous motives; and we entitle practical all that which is *possible* through freedom. But experience also discloses that this power of reason gives rise to prescriptions of obligation (*Sollen*). Hence we pass here from a power to a duty. These two notions are already intimately connected.

The rationality of these laws confers on them both universality and necessity, and constitutes their objectivity. Such laws (also called practical laws) are of two sorts: pragmatic and moral. In a certain sense, this distinction prefigures the one Kant later establishes between hypothetical and categorical imperatives (though not quite perfectly, since in the Canon of Pure Reason Kant does not yet have the notion of a true categorical imperative, both synthetic and a priori).

Pragmatic laws are rules of prudence prescribed by reason, through which we may attain happiness and satisfy our impulses. They do not command. They simply advise us what we must do if we want to be happy. Only experience can tell us which impulses want to be satisfied and what techniques must be employed to satisfy them. Thus, these imperatives are based on empirical principles. Reason only intervenes to achieve a harmony among the several means which promote the empirical end of happiness. In this role, reason places itself in the service of sensibility, yet without thereby subordinating itself to it. The rational being, which submits itself to pragmatic laws, only directs itself to the satisfaction of sensuous needs to the extent that reason advises it, and judges such satisfaction useful in promoting happiness. For its own good, sensibility is, so to speak, under the tutelage of prudential reason.

By contrast, *moral laws* absolutely command the way we must act if we would make ourselves worthy of happiness. This is not an empirical end, but one given completely a priori by reason. Reason establishes the end and shows what must be done to realize it. Nevertheless, reason is not in this way subjected to a goal which is alien to it. "[The] pure moral laws . . . determine completely *a priori* (without regard to empirical motives, that is, to happiness) what is and is not to be done, that is, [they] determine *the employment of the freedom of a rational being in general.*"[6] This is an especially interesting passage, since it reveals the character of that freedom which realizes itself by prescribing an end which is just its own end. More precisely, given that we must distinguish between practical freedom and moral freedom at this level, we can say that the positing of the pure moral law appears as the supreme exaltation of a practical freedom which prescribes what a rational being, insofar as it is endowed with moral freedom, must do to realize the end which it a priori and of necessity posits.

The existence of such a pure practical employment of reason is attested by experience: we establish by experience that we are subject to moral imperatives; moreover, we establish by experience that we have it in us to obey these imperatives. Duty is always connected to ability. At the same time, I encounter this ability *in itself,* not in discrete acts, for experience cannot tell us whether or not there are human acts which could be genuinely moral. "Pure reason, then, contains, not indeed in its speculative employment, but in that practical employment which is also moral, principles of the *possibility of experience,* namely, of such actions as, in accordance with moral precepts, *might* be met with in the *history* of mankind."[7]

The practical employment of reason requires a "canon"[8]—that is, a set of a priori principles which make such employment possible and legitimate. This canon must include a synthetic a priori judgment which expresses the a priori synthesis of the will and the pure moral law. But how can this law, which regulates how I should act in order to make myself worthy of happiness, impose itself on my will? It could not do so if happiness could not be realized in proportion to the morality of an act. Because of natural laws, however, the conjunction between happiness and virtue, which defines the idea of the highest good, cannot be realized in the sensible world. It is possible only in a future life in an intelligible world, where it will be guaranteed by a supreme reason—God. "Thus without a God and without a world invisble to us now but hoped for, the glorious ideas of morality are indeed objects of approval and admiration, but not *springs* of purpose and action. For they do not fulfil in its completeness that end which is natural to every rational being and which is determined *a priori,* and rendered necessary, by that same pure reason."[9] Kant will even affirm that the moral laws cannot be commandments if they do not join the highest good to their prescriptions a priori as a necessary consequence, "and thus carry with them *promises* and *threats.*"[10] Hence it is clear that the moral laws are not absolutely pure: they impose themselves on the subject only insofar as his sensibility is affected by threats and promises. The moral imperative, therefore, is not properly speaking a categorical imperative, synthetic and a priori, since it is not absolutely unconditioned, and can be expressed in the form of a hypothetical imperative: If you desire the highest good, act as you ought to act. If the subject is determined to place himself under the moral law only by virtue of the idea of sanction or reward or chastisement, his intention will always be impure. He will act in conformity with duty, but not because of duty. Thus, the conditions which were intended to ground the synthetic character of the synthesis of will and pure legislation are set out in such a way that they destroy that synthesis itself. The relation of the will to the moral law is in reality analytic, since the desire for the means is included analytically in the desire for the end. In the Transcendental Doctrine of Method, it is the highest good which grounds morality.

Practical laws manifest rational causality. The action of the human will always implies a *Sollen.* When I say "I want," that signifies that I form—freely, by my intellect—the concept of an end. Such a concept is included in the notion of the ought-to-be. I represent to myself the action I ought to perform, and this representational cause of the act breaks out of the order of natural causality. Duty loses all its significance if one simply considers the course of nature. "This *'ought'* expresses a possible action the ground of which cannot be anything but a mere concept; whereas in the case of a merely natural action the ground must always be an appearance."[11] The causality of a concept does not necessarily belong to it intrinsically; instead the concept is laid down contingently as a determining principle for the will. In other words, the bond which unites the concept and the

causality is synthetic, not analytic. Reason establishes a given concept as a principle of action, and by so doing confers causal power on
it. Thus the ought-to-be manifests rational causality, even when the
maxim of action seems to arise from sensibility.

Whether what is willed be an object of mere sensibility (the pleasant) or
of pure reason (the good), reason will not give way to any ground which is
empirically given. Reason does not here follow the order of things as they
present themselves in appearance, but frames for itself with perfect spontaneity an order of its own according to ideas, to which it adapts the
empirical conditions, and according to which it declares actions to be
necessary, even although they have never taken place, and perhaps never
will take place. And at the same time reason also presupposes that it can
have causality in regard to all these actions, since otherwise no empirical
effects could be expected from its ideas.[12]

"While we thus through experience know practical freedom to
be one of the causes in nature, namely, to be a causality of reason in
the determination of the will, transcendental freedom demands the
independence of this reason—in respect of its causality, in beginning a series of appearances—from all determining causes of the
sensible world. Transcendental freedom is thus, as it would seem,
contrary to the law of nature, and therefore to all possible experience; and so remains a problem."[13] This passage from the Doctrine
of Method seems to reinforce three fundamental ideas. First, it establishes a clear distinction between practical and transcendental
freedom. It is interesting that the sensible world provides the point
of orientation permitting us to grasp this distinction. Transcendental
freedom is characterized by an absolute independence from this
world, to the point that it seems to contradict the laws of nature.
Practical freedom, on the other hand, is so to speak inserted into
nature itself to free us from determination by the strictly sensuous.
Whereas in the first case rational causality is absolutely independent
of *all* natural causes, in the second case, reason, with regard to its
causality, is presented as "*one of the natural causes.*" From this first idea
two consequences follow. One is clearly expressed in the text itself:
transcendental freedom—radically heterogeneous with the sensible
world—cannot in any way be an object of experience, and remains
thus a *problem*. Practical freedom, by contrast, remains in close relation to the sensible world. It can perhaps be evidenced and even

known by experience. Hence, the problem of the reality of transcendental freedom cannot call the pure practical employment of reason into question, since I grasp that employment undeniably through psychological experience. "The question of transcendental freedom is a matter for speculative knowledge only, and when we are dealing with the practical, we can leave it aside as being an issue with which we have no concern." [14] But then, second, the fact of practical freedom reveals nothing about the reality of transcendental freedom. These two types of freedom are inscribed in two radically heterogeneous spheres: one is a *problematic concept of reason,* the other a *fact demonstrated by experience.*

One conclusion is unavoidable: the doctrine of morality presented in the Doctrine of Method is not congruent with the assertions in the Dialectic. As we have already seen, the thesis of the third antinomy presents a practical interest, insofar as the freedom of a thinking being appears properly as one of the "foundation stones of morals and religion." We also know that the text of the Doctrine of Method is older than that of the Dialectic. [15] Thus we must acknowledge that Kant's thinking on this matter evolved in a manner we can discern even within the *Critique of Pure Reason.* In the Dialectic, transcendental freedom is presented as one of the ingredients of practical freedom. There, practical freedom is not considered an empirical concept, but a "mainly empirical" one, [16] thus granting that it includes an element inaccessible to experience. This element is both "fundamental" and "problematic": "The practical concept of freedom is based on this *transcendental* idea, . . . [and] in the latter lies the real source of the difficulty by which the *question* [my emphasis] of the possibility of freedom has always been beset." [17] This element is fundamental: practical freedom, which is *"one of the causes in nature"* [18] capable of determining the will according to rational principles, nevertheless presupposes that there is in the will "a causality . . . which can therefore begin a series of events *entirely of itself,"* [19] *"independently of . . . natural causes."* [20] Notice that the ambiguity of practical freedom stems from the intermediate position it seems to occupy between nature, into which it is in some manner inserted, and transcendental freedom, on which it is grounded. "The denial of transcendental freedom must, therefore, involve the elimination of all practical freedom." [21]

As we have already seen, the concept of cosmological freedom is a problematic concept. Thus it is not surprising to discover certain difficulties at the very center of practical freedom, which it inherits precisely because its own constitution includes a problematic element. For the question of the (logical) possibility of transcendental freedom becomes at the same time the question of the possibility of practical freedom. But we know how that problem was resolved. Thus, practical freedom is possible,[22] and its reality is demonstrated by experience. The psychological concept of freedom is no empty concept. It has real content. Nevertheless, an empty space remains within those concepts which transcendental freedom, if its objective reality can be established, will eventually occupy. Hence, a nonempirical element at the center of practical freedom remains unexplicated—and inexplicable.

Still, the foregoing analysis raises a problem. In the Doctrine of Method the fact of practical freedom reveals nothing about the reality of transcendental freedom. This should be no cause for surprise, since the two concepts were radically independent of one another. But it is no longer so in the Dialectic: from now on practical freedom includes transcendental freedom as its ground.

If it is true, as Kant claims, that the problem of cosmological freedom brings with it the question of the possibility of practical freedom, then we must admit that the reality of practical freedom is not the object of any apodictic certainty. And if it were not true, then Kant would not have asserted that the denial of transcendental freedom would eliminate all practical freedom. Doubtless one could object that the reality of practical freedom gives us a preliminary indication that the problem of the third antinomy is not insoluble. But then why doesn't the affirmation of practical freedom entail a correlative affirmation of transcendental freedom? An important passage from the Doctrine of Method provides an answer to this question. According to Kant we can always ask ourselves "whether reason is not, in the actions through which it prescribes laws, itself again determined by other influences, and whether that which, in relation to sensuous impulses, is entitled *freedom,* may not, in relation to higher and more remote operating causes, be *nature* again."[23] This passage introduces us to the heart of the problem and, at the same time, to its solution—but it is a self-defeating solution. Practical freedom, as a *relative* freedom situated in an intermediate position between nature and transcendental freedom, may in reality be a mere chimera—a pseudofreedom. Perhaps a sensuous determinism is hidden behind practical freedom, so that we too quickly christen as freedom what is in fact only nature. Certainly experience testifies that rational causality manifests a certain independence of my will from sensuous impulses, but "there is no way of knowing whether, originally and metaphysically, reason itself, in the very action by which it prescribed to the will the law of an action independent of sensuous impulses, acted with equal independence from the sensuous." [24] Does this not account for that reticence with which Kant expresses himself on the subject of rational causality: "That our reason has causality, or that we *at least represent it to ourselves* [my emphasis] as having causality [*wenigstens wir uns eine dergleichen an ihr vorstellen*], is evident from the *imperatives* which in all matters of conduct we impose as rules upon our active powers"? [25] "Now, in view of these considerations, let us take our stand, and regard it as *at least possible* [*wenigstens als möglich annehmen*] for reason to have causality with respect to appearances." [26] A freedom revealed only in experience risks being nothing more than an illusion. Under such conditions, what could authorize us to affirm the reality of intelligible freedom? Practical freedom remains too closely tied to nature (with which it can even be confused) to permit us to raise ourselves above nature to the realm where true freedom reigns. Thus at the outset of this analysis, practical freedom was laid down as an empirical fact; but at the end of this analysis, we can affirm that Kant never confuses the experience of freedom with freedom itself.

These passages from the *Critique of Pure Reason* announce the subsequent orientation of Kant's thought. Practical freedom is torn, so to speak, between the pole of nature and the pole of intelligible freedom. And remarkably, the concept, too, divides into two elements: one which will rejoin the domain of nature, and one (which will properly retain the name practical freedom) which will be conjoined with transcendental freedom. The first will be connected with the pragmatic laws; the second, with the pure moral law, or the categorical imperative. Practical freedom will become genuinely moral freedom.

Kant had not yet perceived that the pure moral law is apprehended as a fact of reason and not as a practical, empirical fact. Such a practical law remains imperfectly defined in its basic character. Is it an absolutely pure moral law? No, for it is based on the idea

of the highest good, and does not truly command in an unconditioned way. Still, certain passages lead us to think that Kant already
glimpsed something which might be an autonomy of the will: did he
not assert that reason *determines itself,* and determines the will to act
by virtue of a *pure,* entirely a priori moral law, which commands in
an absolutely *unconditioned* manner?

3   *Intelligible Character*

As an application of transcendental freedom to the human will, intelligible character effects the synthesis of practical freedom and
transcendental freedom. It introduces into practical freedom the
element of transcendental freedom which precludes our reducing
the psychological concept of freedom to a purely empirical concept.
To start with, we must attend to the very expression "intelligible
character" and justify the meaning this nomenclature carries. Strictly
speaking, character designates a law, rather than a thing. "Every efficient cause must have a *character,* that is, a law of its causality, without which it would not be a cause."[1] This character will be called
empirical or intelligible, according to whether it involves an empirical or an intelligible causality. Everything in nature, insofar as it is
endowed with causality, has empirical character;[2] in the sensible
world, each efficient cause has a universal and invariable law of its
own causality, which expresses its nature and according to which it
determines one effect rather than another. Man is no exception; to
the extent that he is an appearance in the sensible world, he necessarily has an empirical character. But on the other hand, he is the
only being in nature to whom we have any reason (*Grund*) for attributing an intelligible character, because only in him do we discover an intelligible power (reason) endowed with an intelligible (rational) causality.[3] Only a being endowed with intelligible causality,
or more precisely—since Kant names intelligible "whatever in an
object of the senses is not itself appearance"[4]—only a phenomenal
being, which is not *merely* an appearance, can have an intelligible
character. Thus, in the rational subject we would have "first, an *empirical character,* whereby its actions, as appearances, stand in thoroughgoing connection with other appearances in accordance with
unvarying laws of nature. . . . Secondly, we should also have to allow
the subject an *intelligible character,* by which it is indeed the cause of
those same actions [in their quality] as appearances, but which does

33

not itself stand under any conditions of sensibility, and is not itself appearance."[5]

Notice that Kant does not yet say explicitly what he will affirm later on in the second *Critique*, namely, that it is the rational subject itself which, in relation to the moral law, gives itself a particular character. Delbos remarks, "Here we are dealing with an unknowable, intelligible *thing*, not an intelligible *action*."[6] At first, character is presented as an *idea of reason*—a regulative idea which serves as a principle for explicating human action; moreover, it is directly connected to the cosmological problem of freedom. In the second *Critique* Kant takes up this theory once again and adapts it to the demands of morals: character is now the result of a nontemporal *choice*, according to which the subject freely determines the totality of his actions in the sensible world. Finally, in *Religion within the Limits of Reason Alone*, Kant specifies the *contents* of this choice. These are the three essential stages we can distinguish in the development of the theory of the intelligible character.

The freedom of reason is presented under two aspects: a negative aspect, insofar as it is made manifest by "independence of empirical conditions," and a positive aspect, insofar as it is a "power of originating a series of events."[7] Here we reencounter the two aspects which we had already discerned in practical freedom. The causality of freedom there was always *relative*, since its spontaneity was measured in relation to the determinism of sensuous impulses. But here rational causality is envisaged as *absolutely* spontaneous. Whereas the former was witnessed to by experience, this latter is grasped by that "apperception"[8] (see pp. 12–13) through which man knows himself as an intelligible object. The nonempirical element of practical freedom is apprehended in an apperception.

Reason's absolute spontaneity is defined no differently than transcendental freedom itself. Intellectual causality, like all intelligible causality, is situated *outside* the series of empirical conditions; that is, it is *nontemporal*.

> Now this acting subject would not, in its intelligible character, stand under any conditions of time; time is only a condition of appearances, not of things in themselves. In this subject no *action* would *begin* or *cease*. . . . Inasmuch as it is *noumenon*, nothing *happens* in it; there can be *no change* [my emphasis] requiring dynamical determination in time. . . . No action begins *in* this active being itself; but we may yet quite correctly say that the active being *of itself* begins its effects in the sensible world.[9]

In this way, the assertion that the character of every efficient cause is defined by the law of its own causality quite naturally leads Kant to think of the human will as governed by an *immutable* law. "The law of the causality of a cause," Jean Nabert says, "led Kant to impose the immutability of law on the human will, as a species of intelligible character."[10] Must we conclude, then, that Kant renounces this aspect of the theory of character when, in the *Religion,* he admits the possibility of a "conversion" of the will? We should notice that the immutability of the thing in itself, and of its character, is only the immutability defined by relation to alterability in time. Therefore, as Gueroult observes, it is not "a quality intrinsic to the thing in itself, but an external qualification, related to its opposition to time"; as a result "it in no way excludes, in the thing in itself, a movement of free determination."[11] Certainly the first *Critique* hardly emphasizes this alterability (*mobilité*) of freedom, but "the essential thing is that the *germ* of reason's innate [*originaire*] alterability is in no way stifled by any intrinsic inalterability of the thing."[12] Thus, it accords well with the earlier theories when Kant later acknowledges the possibility of a nontemporal conversion within the intelligible character.

Since the idea of freedom is present only in the relation of the intelligible, as a cause, to appearances, as effects, intelligible causality can only be characterized as free to the extent that it determines a cause to produce a sensible effect. There must be a specific relation, therefore, between the intelligible character and the empirical character. Evidently this relation obtains under two aspects which, although indissolubly bound together, must nevertheless be clearly distinguished.

The relation of the intelligible character to the empirical character is, first of all, a *relation of cause to effect.* It is a fundamental relation, since it is precisely here that the idea of freedom appears. The intelligible character, which is the law of the causality of an efficient cause, produces its effects in the sensible world: the causality of reason "is present in all the actions of men at all times and under all circumstances, and is always the same."[13] It is immutable. It does not modify itself, although its appearances are modified. Thus every act of a rational being is "*the immediate effect* of the intelligible character of pure reason."[14] While this intelligible causality must not be envisaged "as only a co-operating agency," since it is rather perfectly "complete in itself [*an sich selbst . . . vollstandig*],"[15] it remains no less true that the effects it produces also derive from sensible causality.

After the solution of the third antinomy, we know there is no contradiction in conceiving the causal power of a subject as both an "empirical concept" and an "intellectual concept," and regarding both "as referring to *one and the same effect*."[16] It follows that the empirical character produces the same effects as the intelligible character: it is "the empirical cause of all [human] actions," considered as appearances.[17] As an intelligible character, it is "constant," even though "its effects . . . appear in changeable forms."[18] Once we have posited this double causality in each single effect, it is easy to see how the intelligible character must be considered the cause of the empirical character. We know empirical character from its manifestation in nature. If we work with appearances, we can, by a simple induction, isolate the law of their sensible causality: "Empirical character must itself be discovered from the appearances which are its effect and from the rule to which experience shows them to conform"[19] Since the same appearances are also the effect of an intelligible character, the latter can properly be called "the *transcendental cause* of their empirical character."[20] As a result, "a different intelligible character [gives] a different empirical character."[21] Nevertheless, Kant does not specify whether the latter results entirely from the former.[22] If we consider the totality of effects produced by man, it does indeed seem that a part of their empirical character remains unrelated to their intelligible character. Man, as a being in nature, possesses forces like those found in inanimate, or merely animal nature. If the entirety of an intelligible character corresponds to an empirical character, the opposite is not necessarily true, since other beings in nature, besides humans, have an empirical character without having an intelligible character. By contrast, if we consider the entirety of (voluntary) human acts in appearances, we seem to have grounds for the affirmation that every empirical character is determined in its totality by an intelligible character: "Reason is the abiding condition [*die beharrliche Bedingung*] of *all* those actions of the will under [the guise of] which man appears. Before ever they have happened, they are *one and all* predetermined in the empirical character. . . . *every* action . . . is the immediate effect of the intelligible character of pure reason."[23] To make use of a spatial metaphor, we may say that the empirical character is coextensive with the intelligible character. In this context it is not inappropriate to speak of the freedom of the empirical character, since it is the effect of the intelligible character, and every effect "may be regarded as free *in respect of* its intelligible cause." [24]

Thus the intelligible character is the cause of the empirical character. But is not the effect the sign of its cause? It should not surprise us then that the relation which unites the two characters is presented as a *relation of sign and thing signified.*

The empirical character can be "known through experience." [25] The intelligible character certainly cannot be grasped in experience immediately, since it is outside the series of appearances. We have no intuition of it, nor any particular concept, but rather only a "general concept." [26] Hence it cannot be known. This indeed is the paradox of Kant's language—that it is precisely the intelligible which escapes the grasp of our intelligence. [27] Yet no sooner has he reaffirmed that the intelligible character is situated beyond the limits of our knowledge than he expresses a certain reserve on just this point. Is not the sign the indication of what is signified? The intelligible character is "completely unknown, save in so far as the empirical serves for its *sensible sign* [*das sinnliche Zeichen*]." [28] The empirical character, "which is no more than the *appearance* [*die Erscheinung*] of the intelligible," [29] would be a "mediating representation" [30] which permits us to grasp the intelligible character itself, through the mediation of experience. Kant emphasizes this mediating role when he calls the empirical character the "*sensible schema* [*das sinnliche Schema*]" [31] of the intelligible character. The schema, or the "sensible concept," [32] allows us to conceive the relation of the intelligible as cause to the sensible as effect. Inasmuch as it is an empirical causality, and therefore at the same time an appearance, the empirical character is homogeneous with the sensible. Inasmuch as it is the law of the causality of an efficient cause (a law we could isolate by induction from the observation of appearances), the empirical character is also an intellectual representation. But these appearances which manifest the empirical character and, over against it, the intelligible character, follow on one another without our ever being able to grasp them in their totality. Hence we cannot claim to win access, through their intercession, to knowledge of the intelligible character. To know this character, we would need the power of grasping it in itself—directly, by an intellectual intuition; but such an intuition is unavailable to us. Thus we must say about intelligible character what we have already said about transcendental freedom: we can think it, but we can never know it. We can work back from the effect to the intelligible cause, but this cause is never more than an idea of reason. "This intelligible character can never, indeed, be immediately known [*unmittelbar gekannt*], for nothing can be perceived except in so far as it appears. It would have to be *thought* in accordance with the empirical character [*den empirischen Charakter gemäss*]—just as we are constrained to think a transcendental object as underlying appearances, though we know nothing of what it is in itself."[33] This character remains an Object = X, of which we can grasp only its effects in the phenomenal order. We do not know it, but "we indicate [*bezeichen*] its nature by means of appearances."[34]

We can think the relation of the intelligible as cause to the sensible as effect, but we cannot know it. In appealing to this essential distinction between thinking and knowing, we can understand why Kant maintains that "our imputations can refer only to the empirical character,"[35] while he elsewhere affirms that the intelligible character is conceived as the "proper ground of . . . imputability."[36] These are not contradictory affirmations.

The intelligible character is a *regulative* idea of reason, which permits us to conceive, in a reasonable being, grounds for our judgments of imputability. These judgments are practical, empirical facts, evident through experience. For example, suppose that a man disrupts society by telling a pernicious lie. Like every appearance, this lie could be explained by starting from the natural causes which have determined it—that is, one could discover the sources of the act in bad education, bad company, bad temperament, and so on (and without overlooking the particular circumstances involved in the actual occurrence). Assuredly, all these causes, while sufficient to determine the act, cannot be imputed to the liar.[37] Yet still we will hold him culpable; we will blame him. For this reason we think we can attribute the act to the causality of reason, considering the latter as a "completely free [*völlig frei*]" cause, "complete in itself [*an sich selbst vollständig*],"[38] which, in spite of all the empirical conditions of the act, could and ought to determine the conduct of the man otherwise. "The action is ascribed to the agent's intelligible character; in the moment when he utters the lie, the guilt is entirely his."[39] This judgment of imputability is a fact of experience and in itself has no apodictic validity; yet it is only thanks to the speculative hypothesis of the intelligible character that we now know that such a judgment is not inconceivable. Thus Kant evokes the fact of experience "in order to *illustrate* this regulative principle of reason by an example of its empirical employment—not, however, to *confirm* it, for it is useless to endeavour to prove transcendental propositions by examples."[40]

The intelligible character, which grounds our judgments of imputability, remains unknowable. As a result, it is impossible for us to know "why in the given circumstances the intelligible character should give just *these* appearances and *this* empirical character."[41] Conversely, it is impossible for us to determine according to the empirical character if a given being acts freely in a particular circumstance. The relation between the two characters remains permanently unspecifiable. It follows that

the real morality of actions, their merit or guilt, even that of our own conduct, thus remains entirely hidden from us. Our imputations can refer only to the empirical character. How much of this character is ascribable to the pure effect of freedom, how much to mere nature, that is, to faults of temperament for which there is no responsibility, or to its happy constitution (*merito fortunae*), can never be determined; and upon it therefore no perfectly just judgments can be passed.[42]

In their underlying intentions, our acts escape us. Since the idea of intelligible character does not even authorize us to affirm the objective reality of freedom, still less can it enable us to discriminate between what in us is nature and what is freedom. Intelligible character is only an idea of reason; it does not inform us about anything.

Conclusion to Part I

Freedom is one of three major problems imposed on man's metaphysical reflection. Kant never stops reminding us of this. "These unavoidable problems set by pure reason itself are *God, freedom,* and *immortality.* The science which . . . is in its final intention directed solely to their solution is [called] metaphysics."[1] But even metaphysics, which exists in man by a natural disposition, has never yet found the royal road to this science. The failure of metaphysics seems to condemn man to ponder his destiny and the meaning of his life without ever being able to provide satisfactory answers to his queries.

If this failure of metaphysics should prove to be definitive, it would be no exaggeration to affirm that man would thereby be plunged into a tragic situation. Indeed, the tragic character of the human condition is already intimated in the declaration which opens the first *Critique.* "Human reason has this peculiar fate that in one species of its knowledge it is burdened by questions which, as prescribed by the very nature [*Natur*] of reason itself, it is not able to ignore, but which, as transcending all its powers [*Vermögen*], it is also not able to answer."[2] This affirmation—one of the most remarkable and fascinating in all Kant's philosophy—clearly indicates that, because of the finitude of human reason, and because of the fatal disproportion between the demands of the *Natur* of reason and the extent of its *Vermögen,* the questions which strike closest to man's heart must remain at once inevitable and insoluble.

Kant's project is to save metaphysics and, with it, its claims about God, freedom, and the soul. But the realization of this project requires that we begin by condemning speculative metaphysics, and denounce once and for all the illusion to which theoretical reason succumbs whenever it claims to know things in themselves. The critique confirms the failure of such metaphysics by disclosing the reasons for it. But it does not stop there, for it also intends to be a propaedeutic to the new metaphysics, which it seeks to ground.

40

Thus, the negative aspect of the critical enterprise carries with it a positive counterpart. If, after all, it is a matter of restoring the claims of the old metaphysics, we should not misrepresent the progress which was accomplished in the first *Critique*. The *Critique* shows that one can neither refute nor prove the existence of God, immortality, and freedom. In addition, it establishes that these ideas are not at all contradictory. If the conflict between nature and freedom had been determined to be real, freedom would have had "to be surrendered in competition with natural necessity";[3] freedom would have had to "yield to the *mechanism of nature.*"[4] By demonstrating that "nature and freedom therefore can without contradiction be attributed to the very same thing, but in different relations,"[5] speculative reason proved that freedom could be thought, "that is to say, the representation of it is at least not self-contradictory."[6] Admittedly the concept of freedom remains empty and problematic. But it is no less true, however, that it is capable of receiving a content. Thus, "if we grant that morality necessarily presupposes freedom . . . as a property of our will; if, that is to say, we grant that it yields practical principles—original principles, proper to our reason—as *a priori data* of reason, and that this would be absolutely impossible save on the assumption of freedom,"[7] then practical reason would grant a "signification" to the concept of freedom, give it a "practical, objective reality," without thereby falling into self-contradiction, since it is still "assured against [the] opposition" of speculative reason.[8] The *Critique* has a positive utility, since it makes possible the extension of practical reason beyond the limits of sensibility. Speculative philosophy appears as a sort of "precursor" of morality, inasmuch as it falls to it "to level the ground, and to render it sufficiently secure for moral edifices of these majestic dimensions,"[9] or again, to "clear the way for practical philosophy."[10]

From this point of view, Kant's philosophy assumes the form of a diptych. He sounds a death knell for speculative metaphysics by inaugurating a metaphysics according to ethics. He restrains the pretensions of speculative reason in order to make an extension of practical reason possible. He limits knowledge in order to leave room for belief. He dispels the false complacency of a reason nourished by illusions in order to be ready to calm the authentic restlessness of a reason which justifiably questions itself about human destiny. In short, he opens to metaphysics a new path beyond the impasse at

which it had found itself. The transcendental idealism of appearances and the objective reality of the intelligible world make up the
two panels of this diptych. "There are two cardinal principles of all
metaphysics," Kant claims, "the ideality of space and time, and the
reality of the concept of freedom." [11] It has not been without purpose
to emphasize the manner in which they are expressed before turning
to the second panel of the diptych.

II *FREEDOM AND MORALITY*

4   The Self-Positing of Freedom: The Autonomy of the Will

The discovery of the idea of the autonomy of the will, in 1785, marks a decisive turn in the development of Kant's thought. He presents this idea as holding a place in practical philosophy analogous to the place the Copernican revolution holds in theoretical philosophy. Yet it also marks the point of departure for a long evolution in his thought. Although it is expressed for the first time in the *Grundlegung,* it appears faintly even in the first *Critique.* At the time of the first *Critique,* however, Kant was not yet in full possession of the idea; instead it is precisely the *absence* of the idea which permits us, in retrospect, to assess the reservations Kant expresses there, as well as the dissonance which obtained then between certain of his claims. The uncertain status of practical freedom, and of the causality of reason, and the extraordinary concept of a pure moral law (to which promises and threats are nevertheless attached), all indicate that the idea of autonomy was in gestation there. Thus it must be seen as the natural fruit of a slow process of maturation, rather than the product of a sudden inspiration. But after all, it is this idea of the autonomy of the will which legitimizes the continued efforts of moral thought to discover a point of balance.

Before going any further, we must determine the precise point at which the idea emerges in Kant's thought. Interestingly, he introduces the concept in the course of quite disparate analyses and under quite different headings. These analyses represent the many different types of approach through which Kant mastered the concept in its different aspects. Hence, it would be unwise to pass directly to an analysis of the concept without first taking care to examine the different contexts in which it emerges. Let us begin by noting that we can discern three essential stages in the progress of Kant's thought: (*a*) the autonomy of the will first appears as a condition of the logical possibility of the categorical imperative; (*b*) in addition, the categorical imperative requires the autonomy of the will as a condition of its transcendental possibility; (c) the objective reality of the will's autonomy is attested to by a fact of reason.

Three principle texts mark these stages: the second and third sections of the *Grundlegung,* and the "Analytic" of the *Critique of Practical Reason.* We will examine each in turn.

Freedom Is the *Ratio Essendi* of the Moral Law

The interest and originality of the second section of the *Foundations of the Metaphysics of Morals* stem in large part from the fact that Kant, even before proving the objectivity of the concept of duty, strives to establish its validity. In order both to illuminate the meaning of the concept of duty and to discover the conditions of the logical possibility of the concept, he presses the analysis he had outlined in the first section further, determining what is required for the concept of duty to be conceived without contradiction. The examination of the judgments of the common conscience demonstrated to Kant that the idea of duty was inextricably tied to that of a good will. In truth these are mere ideas, and their objective reality remains questionable. Certainly we have the idea of a good will, but we do not know whether such a will really exists. In the same way, we have the idea of duty, but we do not know whether duty is real, or merely "a vain delusion and a chimerical concept."[1] Perhaps duty has no relation to human acts. Nevertheless, no one can doubt that it exists in the mind with the force of a demand. Hence it must be possible to specify the meaning of such a demand, even if that meaning should in the process prove to be purely illusory for us. "We *can* at least show what we understand by the concept of duty and *what it means,* even though it remain undecided whether that which is called duty is an *empty concept* or not."[2] Yet an assertion like this must be justified. By indicating how the categorical imperative can be articulated on the basis of the notion of duty, Kant's analysis provides such a justification.

It would be the ruin of morality, according to Kant, to try to base it on experience. The concept of duty is not an empirical concept. The moral law originates in reason completely a priori; thus, it is valid for all rational beings. For a completely rational being, in whom the will is placed under subjective impulses derived from sensibility (motives which do not always conform to the prescriptions of reason), the law presents itself in the form of a *commandment.* The repre-

sentation of an objective principle as something which compels the
will is called an *imperative*. The moral law imposes itself on the completely rational being in the form of a categorical imperative, that is,
an imperative which represents an action as objectively necessary—
as necessary in itself—without regard for any purpose. Such an imperative is opposed in this way to all hypothetical imperatives, which
only enjoin an act insofar as it serves as a means for attaining some
end posed beforehand. While these imperatives may well be called
principles of action, only the categorical imperative is valid as a practical law of the will.[3] Here the first condition of the logical possibility
of the concept of duty becomes clear. The imperative of duty must
impose itself on us in a categorical manner. "If duty is a concept
which is to have significance and actual legislation for our actions, it
can be expressed only in categorical imperatives and not at all in
hypothetical ones."[4] But we must also specify that this first condition is also one which will lead us to the discovery of all the others.
Because it is a categorical imperative, it will be possible to establish
the formula for it by a simple analysis of its concept; in this way, too,
the logical implications of the concept of duty can be introduced.

"If there is to be . . . a categorical imperative . . . it must be one
that . . . [*Wenn es denn also . . . einen kategorischen Imperativ geben soll, so
muss es ein solches sein, das . . .*]"[5] This manner of expression characterizes Kant's intention perfectly and leaves no doubt as to the orientation of his analysis. If the categorical imperative could not even be
conceived, the problem of its transcendental ground would never be
raised. In the first place, therefore, we must enumerate the logical
requirements of such an imperative. And among these the autonomy
of the will figures prominently. Moreover, the idea of autonomy will
provide us with a key to the explanation of the transcendental possibility of the categorical imperative. The deduction of the formula of
the categorical imperative constitutes a work in preparation for the
deduction of the categorical imperative itself.

Kant lists no fewer than five formulas of the categorical imperative, and it would exceed the limits of our study to make a detailed
examination of his analysis of each of these formulas. Instead, our
attention must be concentrated on the formula of autonomy. But if
we consider the overall structure of Kant's text, we cannot help
being struck by the distinctive place the principle of autonomy occupies among the other formulas. It is, assuredly, difficult to identify

these formulas. Kant often speaks as if there were only three, for
certain of them are so intimately connected to others that it sometimes seems they should not be distinguished. The classification of
the formulas suggested by H. J. Paton seems to take account of these
nuances and thus to do justice to the entirety of Kant's text.[6] We
reproduce it here:

Formula I (the formula of the universal law): "Act only according to that
maxim by which you can at the same time will that it should become a
universal law."[7]

Formula Ia (the formula of the law of nature): "Act as though the maxim of
your action were by your will to become a universal law of nature."[8]

Formula II (the formula of the end in itself): "Act so that you treat humanity, whether in your own person or in that of another, always as an end
and never as a means only."[9]

Formula III (the formula of autonomy): Act so that "[your] will through its
maxims could regard itself at the same time as universally lawgiving."[10]

Formula IIIa (the formula of the realm of ends): "Every rational being must
act as if he, by his maxims, were at all times a legislative member in the
universal realm of ends."[11]

    Not all of these formulas assume equal importance. The text
clearly indicates that formulas Ia, II, and IIIa are only subsidiary formulas related to formula I, which Kant designates as the "supreme
law [*oberste Gesetz*]" of an "absolutely good will."[12] "The three afore-
mentioned ways of presenting the principle of morality are fundamentally only so many formulas of the very same law."[13] Hence, formula I is the essential formula of the moral law. "If one wishes to gain
a hearing for the moral law," the subsidiary formulas are quite
useful; but, Kant adds, "it is better in moral evaluation to follow the
rigorous method and to make the universal formula of the categorical imperative the basis: Act according to the maxim which can
at the same time make itself a universal law."[14] All this is clear
enough. Yet a serious difficulty arises when we inquire into the place
which the formula of autonomy—"the third practical principle of
the will"[15]—occupies in the text. Should we consider it as a subsidiary formula? Certainly not, since Kant considers autonomy as "the
supreme principle of morality [*oberste Prinzip der Sittlichkeit*]"[16] and as
"the sole principle of morals."[17] Formulas I and III thus seem to rival
each other in importance. We wish to show that their respective
priorities obtain on distinct and separable grounds.

In the second section of the *Grundlegung,* Kant undertakes a two-fold enterprise. In the first place, even before knowing whether the categorical imperative really exists, he attempts to resolve once and for all the problem of its application. In this perspective it is a matter of determining what sort of duties derive from the moral imperative, and then establishing the rules which should orient our moral conduct. The formula of the universal law (formula I) appears to be at once the *supreme law* from which we can deduce the totality of duties [18] and the *supreme criterion* to which one should refer "in moral evaluation." [19] But applying morality is not the same as grounding it, and Kant's principal objective in the *Grundlegung* is precisely, as the very title of the work indicates, to search for the foundation—the *Grund*—of morality. Two steps will be necessary to attain this objective since, as we know, Kant examines the question of the logical possibility of the categorical imperative before that of its real possibility. In the second place, however, the autonomy of the will appears as the condition of the possibility of morality, as *the supreme condition (oberste Bedingung)* [20] of the harmony of the will with universal practical reason. From this point of view, there can be no doubt that formula III outweighs formula I, and so merits the title "supreme principle of morality." [21]

The privileged position of the principle of autonomy is easily explained when we consider that it alone explicitly expresses the very *essence* of the categorical imperative. It should be necessary, according to Kant, "to indicate in the imperative itself, by some determination which it contained, that in volition from duty the renunciation of all interest is the *specific mark* of the categorical imperative, distinguishing it from the hypothetical. And this is now being done in the third formulation of the principle, i.e., in the idea of the will of every rational being as a will giving universal law." [22] The categorical imperative is founded on no interest whatsoever. It is unconditioned. A law which imposed itself on the will from outside would necessarily imply "some interest as a stimulus or compulsion" and present itself as a hypothetical imperative. [23] By contrast, a sovereign law-giving will is of necessity disinterested, since it submits itself to the law which it has itself instituted. The concept of the categorical imperative includes, as a condition of its own logical possibility, the idea of a universal law-giving will.

It is therefore not a chance question whether Kant showed good judgment in situating the formula of autonomy in the third place.

For to him it is less important to follow an order of necessary deductions than to highlight the supremacy of the principle of autonomy, and precisely by inserting it in the third place—at the synthetic moment par excellence. In fact, the principle of autonomy draws together and concentrates in itself all of the other principles. It is closely tied to the principle of the realm of ends, which can hardly be explained apart from it. It also makes possible a harmony between the principle of submission to a universal law and the principle of the dignity of the human being, considered as an end in itself. For without the principle of an autonomous will, it would be impossible for us to think that a rational being could submit to a universal law without thereby ceasing to be an end in itself. "The will of a rational being must always be regarded as legislative, for otherwise it could not be thought of as an end in itself." [24]

In the second section of the *Grundlegung,* Kant's principal objective is to determine the conditions required in order for the categorical imperative to be conceivable. Kant repeats over and again that he in no way claims to prove, in this text, "that that kind of imperative really exists" [25] ("*and with it* the autonomy of the will"). [26] We do not yet know if the will's autonomy exists. "We showed only through the development of the universally received concept of morals that autonomy of the will is *unavoidably connected* with it, or rather that it is its *foundation* [*Grunde*]." [27] We know what the concept of duty logically implies, we know that it is logically grounded on the idea of an autonomous will, but we do not know whether it has an objective value or is merely an "empty concept." [28] Nevertheless, we are now in a position to approach the question of the transcendental possibility of the concept. And it is the idea of the autonomy of the will, which includes the concept of freedom, that directs us toward the solution of the problem.

The question of the possibility of a hypothetical imperative presents no particular difficulty. Someone who desires a given end desires at the same time the means which would enable him to achieve that end. Willing the means is, in this case, analytically contained in willing the end. The connection between the will and the act commanded by this will is, as a result, analytic, and the obligatory character of such an imperative for the will is easily explained. It is not the same with the categorical imperative, wherein the connection is not analytic but a priori synthetic. It is a priori, since it is not derived from experience; rather, the connection between the act and the will is universal and necessary. It is synthetic, since neither the will's obligation to take the moral law for its maxim, nor the connection of the will's maxim with that law, nor the connection of the will with the act prescribed by that law, is analytically included in a prior will. Kant specifies that the connection of the act to the will is conceivable only to the extent that the will is affected, yet not determined necessarily, by subjective determining causes. Moreover, the moral law could be analytically deduced from the will if that will were perfect, that is, if it could only be determined by the representation of the good.[29] From this we conclude that our will is good enough to allow us to conceive its connection with the moral law, but not good enough to allow us to conceive that connection as analytic. The synthesis is the mark of our finitude, and of the subjective imperfection of our will.

This imperative is an a priori synthetical practical proposition. . . . I connect a priori, and hence necessarily, the action with the will without supposing as a condition that there is any inclination [to the action] (though I do so only objectively, i.e., under the idea of a reason which would have complete power over all subjective motives). This is, therefore, a practical proposition which does not analytically derive the willing of an action from some other volition already presupposed (for we do not have such a perfect will); it rather connects it directly with the concept of the will of a rational being as something which is not contained within it.[30]

The concept of autonomy, as we conceive it, is also a priori synthetic, for we can only posit the concept through the synthesis of a good will with a universal law. The question of its possibility cannot be distinguished from the question of the possibility of the concept of a categorical imperative. How is an a priori synthetic practical proposition possible? We should note that the categorical imperative cannot be found in experience. Hence, we must examine the question of its possibility completely a priori. And this examination should permit us to establish that possibility, not merely to explain it (as was the case for the synthetic a priori judgments which ground the knowledge of nature and which then are encountered in experience).

The solution to this problem is outlined in the third section of the

Grundlegung and taken up again in the *Critique of Practical Reason*. Both texts employ the same synthetic method: both begin with the idea of freedom, whose objective reality, from the practical point of view, they prove apodictically, by appealing to the affirmation of the moral law, as a "fact of reason."[31] In truth, the important passages of the *Grundlegung* are not very explicit; certain of them could even lead us to think that freedom is affirmed only as a hypothesis. In fact, the ambiguity of the third section stems from its character as a transition from the first *Critique*, certain conclusions of which it recapitulates, to the second *Critique,* certain affirmations of which it anticipates. In any case, the third section is particularly preoccupied with the question of the real possibility of the categorical imperative. And it is thus preferable, in order not to betray the movement of Kant's thought, to examine that problem first.

The categorical imperative is synthetic a priori. It thus requires a third term, capable of effecting the synthesis between the will of the human being and the universal moral law. This third term is furnished by the concept of freedom. The will is a type of causality which belongs to rational beings. And freedom, understood in a negative sense, is "that property of this causality by which it can be effective independently of foreign causes determining it."[32] Nevertheless, even if the free will did not conform to the laws of nature, we should not believe that it would be therefore removed from all lawfulness. The concept of causality implies the concept of law. A free will which did not act according to a law "would be a pure nothing [*ein Unding*],"[33] and its concept would be contradictory. Isn't the will further defined as the "capacity of acting according to the conception of laws"?[34] The analysis of the free will, far from leading us to replace conformity to the laws of nature (*Gesetzmässig-keit*) with a mere absence of law (*Gesetzlosigkeit*),[35] invites us to determine what that law is according to which it acts. This can only be the moral law, a law which is not *imposed* on the will, since it is *posited* by it. "What else, then, can the freedom of the will be but autonomy, i.e., the property of the will to be a law to itself?"[36] The autonomy of the will, which is nothing else than freedom understood in its positive sense, is opposed both to lawlessness and to heteronomy.[37]

The law of the will is the moral law. "Thus if freedom of the will is presupposed, morality together with its principle follows from it by the mere analysis of its concept."[38] In other words, the imperative, which is an a priori synthetic proposition, "would be analytic if the freedom of the will were presupposed, but for this, as a positive concept, an intellectual intuition would be needed, and here we cannot assume it."[39] We do not know if an autonomous will really exists. Thus, it is impossible for us to deduce the objective reality of the moral law from freedom. Freedom is not the *ratio cognoscendi* of the moral law. We should note, however, that even if it were possible to deduce the principle of morality analytically from freedom, "the principle is nevertheless a synthetical proposition,"[40] since the relation between the will of a finite rational being and the moral law is still synthetic. The principle of morality, which is an a priori synthetic proposition with respect to its transcendental possibility, would be an analytic proposition with respect to its objective reality.

The idea of an intelligible world implied in the *positive* concept of freedom effects the synthesis of the will and the moral law. As the Transcendental Dialectic has already clearly established, the idea of an intelligible world is included in the concept of freedom. We know that the rational being can be considered from two points of view. As an appearance, he belongs to the sensible world and is subject to the laws of natural necessity. As noumenon, he belongs to the intelligible world and is subject to the objective laws of his reason. The *Grundlegung* specifies that these laws based in mere reason are no different from the moral law dictated by practical reason or the autonomous will. Thus, if the human being belonged only to the intelligible world, all his "actions would completely accord with the principle of the autonomy of the pure will."[41] By contrast, if he belonged only to the sensible world, his actions would of necessity conform only to the laws of nature. But we belong to both of these worlds, and, "since the intelligible world contains the ground of the world of sense and hence of its laws,"[42] we are obliged to recognize that we are also subject to the law of the intelligible world, that is, to the moral law. "Thus categorical imperatives are possible because the idea of freedom makes me a member of an intelligible world."[43]

Kant's thought is not easy to grasp at this point. He asserts that the intelligible world grounds the sensible world. This relation, transposed to the realm of the finite rational being, makes possible the a priori synthesis between the will and the law—between a "will affected by . . . sensuous desires" and "the idea of exactly the same will as pure, practical of itself, and belonging to the intelligible world, which according to reason contains the supreme *condition* of the former [sensuously affected] will."[44] It is thus a double relation. On one hand, the pure will which is "a mere member of the intelligible world"[45] *grounds* the will affected by sensuous desires. On the other hand, the moral law establishes "the *ground* of all actions of rational beings"[46] insofar as they, by virtue of their autonomous wills, are members of an intelligible world. This explains how the autonomous will can effect the synthesis of the moral law and the will of a finite rational being.

Pure practical laws have their foundation in "the concept of their existence in the intelligible world, i.e., freedom. . . . For this concept has no other meaning, and these laws are possible only in relation to the freedom of the will."[47] The second *Critique* recapitulates the findings of the *Grundlegung,* but it extends them and completes them by abandoning the clear distinction between the negative and the positive concepts of freedom. The idea of autonomy of the will includes independence with respect to the laws of nature. In the same way that it grounds the autonomy of the will, this independence from natural laws grounds the real possibility of the categorical imperative, since the moral law is possible only so long as I am not subject to strict spatio-temporal determination. Without transcendental freedom, understood as "*independence* from . . . nature generally," and as alone *a priori practical,* "no moral law and no accountability to it are possible."[48] Note that practical freedom is henceforth identified with transcendental freedom. In the Doctrine of Method of the first *Critique,* these two types of freedom were clearly distinguished; in the Dialectic, they were united in a fundamental relation; in the second *Critique,* they are identified through the notion of the autonomy of the will.

Freedom is thus at one and the same time a real and a logical condition of the moral law. Apart from freedom, the categorical imperative would be inconceivable and nonsensical ("impossible and absurd").[49] Apart from freedom, the moral law would be a "mere deception of our reason."[50] Put another way, it "would never have been encountered in us,"[51] for freedom is the *ratio essendi* of the moral law, which causes it to be. "Freedom is the condition of the moral law."[52]

This passage from the preface to the second edition of the first *Critique* shows clearly that the fate of morality is inextricably tied to that fate which speculative reason reserves for freedom and the logical possibility of freedom:

> If we grant that morality necessarily presupposes freedom (in the strictest sense) as a property of our will; if, that is to say, we grant that it yields practical principles—original principles, proper to our reason—as *a priori data* of reason, and that this would be absolutely impossible save on the assumption of freedom; and if at the same time we grant that speculative reason has proved that such freedom does not allow of being thought, then the former supposition—that made on behalf of morality—would have to give way to this other contention, the opposite of which involves a palpable contradiction. For since it is only on the assumption of freedom that the negation of morality contains any contradiction, freedom, and with it morality, would have to yield to the mechanism of nature.[53]

In order to dramatize the debate—to make the issues at stake stand out more clearly—Kant hypothetically poses things which we know to be either absurd or nonexistent; he proceeds as if he were not already in possession of the essential and definitive data of his practical philosophy. For Kant, it is no mere presupposition but a well-established position that morality necessarily implies freedom: did he not explicitly affirm, in an earlier work, that "[morality] [*Sittlichkeit*] is possible only through freedom"?[54] On the other hand, the claim that freedom, and with it morality, would have to yield to the mechanism of nature if speculative reason should demonstrate that freedom does not allow of being thought is an absurd hypothesis. It was already disposed of by the fact that the moral law, and with it freedom, is witnessed to by a "fact of reason."[55] Yet the device Kant employs here also enables us to take hold of the strict progress of his philosophy. Before proving that freedom is the condition of the moral law—and in particular the condition of its logical possibility—was it not necessary to show that freedom itself was logically possible, that there was no contradiction between freedom and nature, that freedom itself was not self-contradictory? These are the terms in which the first *Critique* poses the problem of freedom; and, as the second *Critique* explains, the fact of reason indicates that the problem effectively *had* to be resolved as it was—that is, in a positive sense.

The Moral Law Is the *Ratio Cognoscendi* of Freedom

In order of existence, freedom is prior to the moral law, as its *ratio essendi*. But in order of knowledge, the moral law is first: it is the *ratio cognoscendi* of freedom. "It is therefore the moral law, of which we become immediately conscious . . . , which leads directly to the concept of freedom."[56] That we are conscious of the moral law is an indisputable fact attested by the common conscience. But by itself it neither preserves us from error and illusion nor guarantees that duty and the moral law are not empty, chimerical concepts. If Kant had been content with the affirmation in the second *Critique* that "the consciousness of this fundamental law may be called a fact of reason,"[57] we would be no further than we were at the end of the second section of the *Grundlegung,* and the problem of the objectivity of freedom would remain intact. But it is not really a problem, for the fact of reason is the law of which we are conscious itself and not merely the consciousness of the law. In other words, if the consciousness of the moral law attains the dignity of a fact of reason, that is because when it occurs, the contents of consciousness present themselves as a fact of reason. "The moral law is given, as an apodictically certain fact, as it were, of pure reason, a fact of which we are a priori conscious."[58]

The apodictic certainty attached to the fact guarantees the objective reality of the moral law, and it thereby reveals to us the first truth from which the entirety of Kant's practical metaphysics issues. It is thus important to examine the texts closely in order to determine the nature of that fact. Certainly the phrase "fact of pure reason [*Factum der reinen Vernunft*]" is a strange expression whose peculiar character did not escape Kant. The word *fact* naturally evokes the facticity of sensuous data. The moral law, we recall, "is not an empirical fact."[59] And its objective reality cannot be cast into doubt "even if it be granted that no example could be found in which it has been followed exactly."[60] To put us on guard against this sort of confusion, Kant over and again expresses the embarrassment he feels at his unusual use of the word *fact.* He affirms that the moral law is given as a "fact, as it were, of pure reason [*Gleichsam als ein Factum*]."[61] But precisely by making us aware of his reservations, he also indicates that he coined this peculiar expression only because it seemed to him the most appropriate expression of his thought. The moral law is a fact of reason—that is, rather than arising through a deduction from previously established truths, it is given to us as an original datum, which we cannot go beyond. Properly speaking, it is an authentic "principle" from which other data can doubtless be deduced but which is not itself derived—"ferreted out"—through any process of reasoning.[62] "The consciousness of this fundamental law *may be called* a fact of reason, *since* one cannot ferret it out from antecedent data of reason, . . . and since it forces itself upon us [*es sich für sich selbst uns aufdringt*] as a synthetic proposition a priori based on no pure or empirical intuition."[63] Our certainty about the moral law is thus immediate rather than discursive or intuitive, yet it resembles sensuous certainty more closely than rational certainty. It is, perhaps, not inappropriate to think that, by repeatedly using the adverb *gleichsam,* in expressions like *"gleichsam als ein Factum"*[64] and *"gleichsam durch ein Factum,"*[65] Kant was as much concerned to bring the fact of reason and the empirical fact together as to distinguish them. What is essential is the facticity of the moral law—the fact that reason gives us an immediate datum, which imposes itself by itself and not through any rational derivation, even while, on the other hand, this datum cannot be ferreted out from any experience, since it is necessary and a priori.[66] Taking all of these considerations into account, no other expression would be more appropriate than *Factum der Vernunft.*

Consciousness of the moral law is thus an absolutely primary fact founded on neither practical nor speculative knowledge. This is doubtless Kant's meaning when, in an astonishing formula, he asserts that moral laws are necessary as "practical *postulates.*"[67] The moral law is an absolute principle. It could be the object of no deduction; moreover, it requires no deduction. "Thus the objective reality of the moral law can be proved through no deduction, through no exertion of the theoretical, speculative, or empirically supported reason."[68] The moral law has no criterion besides itself: it is its own standard. "It imposes itself *axiomatically.*"[69] It is "given . . . from within."[70] Nor need its objective reality be grounded on anything beyond itself, since it "is an axiom,"[71] and "it is firmly established of itself."[72]

This moral principle, which requires no deduction and "no justifying grounds,"[73] serves itself as a principle of the deduction of the power of freedom, which it "shows to be not only possible but actual

in beings which acknowledge the law as binding upon them." [74] Freedom is deduced from the moral law; it is the object of a demonstration. Therefore, it is discursively certain and cannot be likened to the
moral law as a fact of reason. But what does this proof of freedom
gain us? Does it acquire the same apodictic certainty which characterizes the fact of the law? The question is even sharper since Kant
specifies that freedom "cannot be demonstrated *directly*." [75] Certainly the law imposes itself on all rational beings as an ineluctable
moral demand; and we must admit that "if I ought to do something,
I must be able to do it." [76] Yet perhaps the nature of the "therefore"
in the celebrated formula, "You ought, *therefore* you can," [77] surrep-
titiously introduces sufficient uncertainty to make us doubt the objectivity of freedom. Is the movement from the affirmation of a duty
to the affirmation of an ability legitimate? Quite succinctly, do we
have an irrefutable proof here? We cannot escape the importance of
this question, for if we recall that for Kant the reality of freedom
constitutes one of the "two pivots," [78] or one of the "two cardinal
principles," [79] of all metaphysics, we must grant that "the highly consistent structure" [80] of the system is put at risk.

   In this question the painstaking evolution of Kant's philosophy is
fully justified. By showing that the concept of freedom is not contradictory, by proving that freedom constitutes the condition of the
(logical and transcendental) possibility of the moral law, by indicating that the presence of the law in us is evident as a fact of reason,
Kant provides firm support for his proof of freedom. To underscore
the specific character of the proof, we must never lose sight of the
fact that it rests on the fundamental relation which unites freedom
and the moral law. "A rational being's character of possessing, in a
general manner, freedom of the will (that is, of being independent of
natural impulses) cannot be directly demonstrated as a causal principle, but only *indirectly* by its consequences, insofar as it contains the
foundation of the possibility of the categorical imperative." [81] The fact
that it is demonstrated indirectly indicates that we cannot grasp the
power of freedom in itself but merely by virtue of its character as the
foundation, the *ratio essendi,* of the moral law. Apart from freedom,
the moral imperative would be "impossible and absurd." [82] It would
be absurd to maintain the presence of this imperative in us but then
to refuse to admit the existence of its condition. The method of
going back from the conditioned to the condition is a method of

demonstration no less rigorous for being indirect. Indeed, the formula, "You ought, therefore you can," acquires all its significance from it, for it addresses itself to a rational being, to a sensible being living in a world that is not absurd. Silhouetted against the backdrop of the deduction of freedom is the question of meaning itself—the question of the meaning of the world, of the meaning of human fate, of human good sense. We *must* admit freedom because the practical law is real. In the words of B. Rousset, "At issue here is both a logical necessity which forbids us from contradicting ourselves and a transcendental necessity which obliges us to suppose that which makes the law possible." [83] In a world without meaning or in the mind of a fool, no such necessity would impose itself. Indeed, reason's own interest is deeply involved in the problem of freedom since that problem goes straight to the existence of reason itself.

Thus the concept of freedom, which speculative reason had posited as being noncontradictory but which nevertheless remained empty, problematic, indeterminate, and merely limiting, acquires an objective, positive, and determinate reality through the moral law. Still, we have neither a sensible nor an intellectual intuition of freedom, and we must not believe that the moral law makes up for this absence in order to provide a theoretical determination of freedom. The original disclosure of freedom through the apodictic law of practical reason conveys no extension of our knowledge in the theoretical realm. And while we must speak of a certain knowledge of freedom, we can only do so by appealing to the mixed concept of "practical knowledge." [84] Having arisen from the practical law, our knowledge of freedom preserves the stamp of its origin: it acquires an "exclusively practical" significance;[85] and if it receives objective reality "from a practical point of view," [86] "it is not for the purpose of the theoretical but for that of the merely practical use of reason." [87] That is, freedom finds itself invested with an objective reality in no way theoretical, but merely practical.[88] Thus one can speak of a practical understanding of freedom which does not pertain to nature but to the possibility and reality of this freedom. "Freedom, however, among all the ideas of speculative reason is the only one whose possibility we know [*wissen*] a priori. We do not understand [*einzusehen*] it, but we know it as the condition of the moral law which we do know." [89] The moral law is freedom's unique and irreplaceable credential. It would be inadequate to observe merely that the moral law "for the first time . . . gives objective reality to this concept [of free-dom],"[90] and that through it an idea of speculative reason receives objective reality "for the first time."[91] We must make clear that only the moral law could authorize us to view ourselves as "compelled [nötigen]" to assume the existence of freedom.[92] For only the moral law was able to overcome the resistances of speculative reason, which the concept of freedom, being such an embarrassment to it, could not fail to raise. "No one would dare introduce freedom into science had not the moral law and, with it, practical reason come and forced this concept upon us."[93] Certainly speculative reason suc-ceeded in demonstrating that freedom could be reconciled with the mechanism of nature, but this by itself was insufficient to overcome the reluctance of a reason concerned above all to explain appear-ances. "Had not the moral law already been distinctly thought in our reason, we would never have been justified in assuming anything like freedom, even though it is not self-contradictory."[94] Apart from freedom, the moral law would never have been discovered in us; but apart from the moral law, freedom would have remained completely unknown. Freedom grounds the moral law. The moral law proves the existence of freedom. The two concepts reciprocally imply each other.[95]

The two concepts are united so indissolubly that granting one necessarily entails granting the other. This is true of freedom, which is so rigorously deduced from the moral law that it acquires an "in-dubitably" objective reality.[96] But it is also true of the moral law, which could itself be deduced from freedom, even though the latter can only be revealed to us through the moral law. In this regard it is significant that at the same time that he declares that the moral law, as a fact of reason, was not deduced, Kant considers it important to specify that the consciousness of freedom does not precede that of the moral law. "The consciousness of this fundamental law may be called a fact of reason, since one cannot ferret it out from antecedent data of reason, such as the consciousness of freedom (for this is not antecedently given)."[97] Of course, no deduction can prove the objec-tive reality of the moral law. But "instead of this . . . deduction [statt der Deduction,[98] an die Stelle dieser Deduction[99]]" we not only found that the moral principle itself serves as the principle of the deduction of the power of freedom, we showed that "if we saw [einsähe] the possi-bility of freedom as an efficient cause, we would see not only the possibility but also the necessity of the moral law as the supreme practical law of rational beings."[100] But we cannot "see [*einzusehen*]" this possibility of freedom.[101] Hence we cannot hope to deduce the moral law from freedom. Such a deduction we know to be useless and impossible.

But if this is the case, is it not paradoxical that the deduction of freedom which begins with the moral law then rebounds and becomes a deduction of the law itself? By justifying the idea of freedom, the moral law satisfied a need of theoretical reason: through it the cosmological idea of freedom, which is indispensable for the complete and coherent employment of speculative reason, found its justification (*Rechtfertigung*) and thereby an unshakable guarantee (*Sicherung*).[102] That the moral law furnishes objective reality to a natural (but problematic) concept of theoretical reason, in the absence of any a priori justification, constitutes a "kind of credential" for it.[103] The justification for freedom provided by the moral law reflects back on the moral law, which in turn is in a certain fashion justified by freedom. But again, we must recognize that the law, after all, is its own justification: the moral law is not "proved [*bewiesen*]"; rather, it "proves its reality [*beweist seine Realität*]."[104]

The coherence of the system is clearly manifest here.[105] The deduction of freedom provides the fundamental element of the Kantian edifice—the keystone which insures the harmony and solidity of its architecture. It also illuminates the close harmony obtaining between the two types of reason. On one hand, it fills out the concept of an unconditioned causality, which speculative reason was required to form without thereby being able to give it any contents. It reassures speculative reason, in Delbos's words, "by testifying that the production of ideas is no less securely grounded for the fact that it inevitably engenders a dialectic in the order of knowledge."[106] On the other hand, it opens up new perspectives on the intelligible world, enabling us to glimpse the possibility of extending our (practical) knowledge to supersensible objects, and "*in accordance with the wish of metaphysics . . .* [passing] beyond the limits of all possible experience."[107] In this way the significance of one of Kant's fundamental assertions becomes clearer: "The concept of freedom, in so far as its reality is proved by an apodictic law of practical reason, is the keystone of the whole architecture of the system of pure reason and even of speculative reason."[108]

In the terms set out in this analysis, we can conclude that our knowledge of the unconditionally practical begins with the moral law, not with freedom. At the level of our consciousness, the moral law is naturally first. The consciousness of the moral law is immediate, but we cannot know freedom immediately.[109] Freedom's reality is not "demonstrated directly, but only indirectly, through a mediating principle."[110] We are conscious of freedom through the *mediation* of the moral law, but the *movement* from the moral law to freedom is *immediate:* the moral law "leads *directly* to the concept of freedom."[111]

Moreover, "experience also confirms this order of concepts in us."[112] Kant argues that if a man were ordered, under threat of sudden death, to make a false deposition against an honorable man, he would certainly consider it possible to overcome his love of life and follow the moral law. He would acknowledge that he had the power to make a choice, since he is conscious of what he ought to do, and "he recognizes that he is free—a fact which, without the moral law, would have remained unknown to him."[113]

Kant never doubts the primacy of the moral law: in the order of knowledge the moral law reveals itself to us first, as a fact of reason. On the other hand, the question arises whether this "sole fact [*einzige Factum*]" of reason reveals *only* the moral law.[114] Are not freedom and the moral law, two concepts "so inextricably bound together [*so unzertrennlich verbunden*]"[115] that in reality they form "a single concept [*einzigen Begriff*],"[116] revealed indissolubly at one and the same time? This fact, Kant affirms, is "inextricably bound up [*unzertrennlich verbunden*] with the consciousness of freedom of the will, and actually . . . *identical* with it."[117] The movement from the moral law to freedom—an unmediated movement granting freedom a discursive certainty—seems here to yield to a pure identification of the two terms. In other words, freedom was not deduced from the fact of reason but was grasped in and through the fact of reason. Should we then consider freedom as enjoying the same facticity which the moral law does? This possibility, which appears as a doubt about the deduction of freedom from the law, may also shed new light on the notion of a fact of reason, at least in the context where it originally appears. "This Analytic proves that pure reason can be practical, i.e., that of itself and independently of everything empirical it can determine the will. This it does through a fact [*Factum*] wherein pure reason shows itself [*sich beweist*] actually [*in der That*] to be practical. This fact is *autonomy* in the principle of morality by which reason determines the will to action [*That*]."[118] As this passage indicates, the fact of reason reveals the presence in us of an autonomous, pure practical reason which posits the moral law. Moreover, it is less a fact given to reason than reason itself considered as a fact. Thus the phrase "fact of reason" receives a double justification, for in this fact, that which is given to our reason is just reason itself.

The objective reality of a pure will or of a *pure practical reason* (they being the same) is given in the moral law a priori, *as it were by a fact.* . . . In the concept of a will, however, the concept of causality is already contained; thus in that of a pure will there is [*contained*] the concept of causality with freedom, i.e., of a causality not determinable according to natural laws and consequently not susceptible to any empirical intuition as proof. Nevertheless, it completely justifies its objective reality in the pure practical law a priori.[119]

Pure practical reason, the autonomy of the will, and the moral law are three concepts so intimately connected that their objective reality is revealed in one and the same fact. The moral law is "the *sole fact* of pure reason, which by it proclaims itself as originating law (*sic volo, sic iubeo*)."[120] Nevertheless, even here it seems that Kant preserves a certain priority for the law, since, as he never tires of emphasizing, it is "in the moral law [*im moralischen Gesetze; in dem reinen praktischen Gesetze*]" that the objective reality of a pure practical reason is given a priori,[121] and in which the concept of free causality a priori justifies its objective reality. After all, the moral law is the *ratio cognoscendi* of freedom.

In the foregoing analysis it is plain that Kant presents the assertion of the objective reality of freedom from two distinctly different perspectives. Sometimes freedom is known as a fact of reason; sometimes it is deduced directly from a fact of reason. The fact that the priority of the moral law in the order of knowledge is recognized in both cases diminishes the difference in the two concepts without thereby suppressing it altogether. But perhaps it is not wrong to wish to suppress a difference which may not even exist. Does not Kant himself maintain these two apparently divergent positions without ever acknowledging the least incompatibility between them? Does he not present them together in the Analytic without worrying whether there might be any contradiction between them? Without a doubt! But, sadly, we know how fragile this sort of argument is; at the very least it is incumbent on us to inquire whether a reconciliation might not be possible after all. In any case, the facticity of the law cannot be construed according to exactly the same model as the facticity of freedom, even though there can be no doubt that they pertain to one and the same fact. The moral law requires no deduction *because* it is a fact of reason. Freedom, on the other hand, requires a deduction *even though* it is a fact of reason. Is it not perhaps the case that freedom is deduced from a fact of reason in a manner so *immediate* that it is nearly identical with that fact? This would explain how Kant was able to maintain this twofold perspective without jeopardizing the coherence of his system. Rather than speak of his vacillation, as by turns he affirms and then denies the facticity of freedom,[122] we are tempted to adopt the position of Fichte, who, instead of unmasking a contradiction, made bold to assert that "when Kant deduces Freedom from the consciousness of the moral law, he means to say that the manifestation of Freedom is an unmediated fact of consciousness which must not be otherwise deduced."[123] But is it legitimate to reconcile the deduction of freedom with the facticity of freedom in this way? We do not think so. A fact is not deduced. It posits itself. It imposes itself. Freedom must be deduced; and if it should turn out that it is a fact, that is doubtless by virtue of the unmediated connection which joins it to the moral law. The facticity of the law is communicated to freedom as if by osmosis, just as the deduction of freedom indirectly becomes a deduction of the law itself. But it is always through the law that we take hold of freedom. The order of concepts which Kant describes[124] not only indicates that the knowledge of the moral law precedes that of freedom, it indicates that the facticity of freedom follows the deduction of freedom.

Whatever the status of this facticity, it cannot be questioned that Kant considered freedom a fact. Although the main passages in the second *Critique* may seem less than fully explicit on the point, Kant's position leaves no room for doubt. Far from renouncing it, he reiterates it in the third *Critique*, albeit from a slightly different perspective and with certain new accents. There, freedom "is the only one of all the ideas of pure reason whose object is a thing of fact [*Thatsache*] and to be reckoned under the *scibilia*,"[125] for it is the only one which "proves [its] reality in experience." [126] This assertion must be acknowledged, despite its isolated context and its somewhat strange sound. But in order to avoid confusion, we must recall that the concept of freedom is not at all "an empirical concept" [127] but an idea of reason. To speak more precisely, it is "a concept of reason, whose object can be met with nowhere in experience." [128] We have no sensuous intuition of freedom, and it would be hopeless to attempt "to prove it from certain alleged experiences of human nature." [129] Moreover, we could hardly prove freedom "from experience, since experience reveals to us only the law of appearances and consequently the mechanism of nature, the direct opposite of freedom." [130] If, therefore, the reality of freedom may be "exhibited . . . in experience," [131] it can only be done indirectly, since freedom, which certainly cannot be found in nature, nevertheless manifests itself through the effects it produces in nature. Freedom "establishes its reality *in actions* as a fact," [132] insofar as these acts fall under the jurisdiction of the moral law and thereby effectively imply that there is a free causality. In the last analysis, it is through the mediation of the moral law that freedom proves its reality. The reality of freedom, "regarded as . . . a particular kind of causality (of which the concept, theoretically considered, would be transcendent), may be exhibited *by means of practical laws* of pure reason, and conformably to this, in actual actions [*in wirklichen Handlungen*], and consequently, in experience." [133] This justifies the inclusion of freedom among "things of fact [*res facti*]" rather than among "things of faith." By saying this Kant does not mean to suggest that experience proves the reality of freedom. What we grasp in experience is not freedom itself but the actual actions which exhibit freedom. In this sense, we can affirm that freedom is not a fact *of* experience but a fact *in* experience. Although placed "outside the world," it nevertheless "acts on the world," producing sensible effects in it. [134] Yet these effects never furnish a proof of its reality. "There are indeed some things in human reason which no experience can make known to us; but yet their reality and truth is proved by effects which are presented in experience. . . . These include the concept of freedom and the law of the categorical . . . imperative which emanates from it." [135]

The third *Critique* presents the problem of the reality of freedom from a new perspective, which contrasts with that adopted by Kant in the second *Critique*. Hence we must avoid simply assimilating the

res facti into the *factum rationis.* In this respect, one passage from the
second *Critique* seems particularly significant. Here we see Kant ad-
dressing the problem in terms quite like those which he utilizes in
the third *Critique,* yet we also see how the movement of his thought
is very different.

It was a question of whether in an actual case and, as it were, by a fact,
one could prove that certain actions presupposed such an intellectual,
sensuously unconditioned, causality, regardless of whether they are actual
or only commanded, i.e., objectively and practically necessary. In actions
actually given in experience as events in the world of sense we could not
hope to meet with this connection, since causality through freedom must
always be sought outside the world of sense in the intelligible. But things
which are not sensuous are not given to our perception and observation.
Thus nothing remained but that perhaps an incontrovertible, objective
principle of causality could be found which excluded every sensuous condition from its determination, i.e., a principle in which reason does not
call upon anything else as the determining ground of the causality but
rather by that principle itself contains it, thus being, as pure reason,
practical of itself. This principle, however, needs no search and no in-
vention, having long been in the reason of all men and embodied in their
being. It is the principle of morality.[136]

In the second *Critique* the fact of reason is a *principle* from which
we can demonstrate freedom synthetically. It is an a priori given: the
immediate consciousness of the existence of the moral law in us. It is
"an apodictically certain fact, . . . even if it be granted that no example could be found in which it has been followed exactly."[137] It
reveals to us the *autonomy* of pure practical reason, which poses the
fundamental principle of morality "by which reason determines the
will to action."[138] In the third *Critique* this movement is reversed.
Instead of beginning with the moral law and the commandment
which the law imposes on us to perform a particular act in accordance with its own prescriptions, it begins with real acts, effective
and identifiable in nature and susceptible to moral characterization.
From these real acts, which we consider in terms of the commands
of the moral law (but without thereby being in a position to judge
whether they fulfill these commands), we work back *analytically* to
the freedom which they manifest empirically. This does not constitute a rigorous demonstration (*démonstration*) but rather an illustra-
tion (*monstration*). The human being "experiences" freedom through

certain acts.[139] But this freedom is not only the freedom of autonomous reason in posing the moral law; it is also the freedom of the evil
will which freely chooses to transgress the law. The first movement
is more rigorous, since it is grounded on a supersensible fact and
provides an a priori proof of freedom, while the second movement
gains support from sensuous experience, which illustrates freedom a
posteriori, without as a result being able to claim to demonstrate its
reality. On the other hand, the second of these two strategies undeniably has the greater import, for it leads us to a notion of freedom
which encompasses numerous disparate aspects of human freedom.
In the second case, the center of gravity has shifted: in the first, the
factum rationis places us before that which is common to *every* rational
being; in the second, we apprehend freedom as a *res facti* only when
we consider nature and sensuous experience, that is, when we consider the arena in which the freedom of a finite rational being has
effects.

The preceding considerations bring us to recognize that freedom
occupies a privileged place among the ideas of pure reason. Over and
again Kant underscores this point. In relation to the other ideas (God
and immortality), the idea of freedom enjoys certain privileges
which pertain to it in ways we can understand according to the twofold perspective we have analyzed. In the first place, to the extent
that it is a fact of reason, or at least a conclusion derived immediately
from a fact of reason, freedom is the object of a practical knowledge.
It is "determinately and assertorically known."[140] "Freedom . . . ,
among all the ideas of speculative reason is the only one [*das einzige*]
whose possibility we know [*wissen*] a priori. We do not [perceive]
[*einzusehen*] it, but we know it as the condition of the moral law
which we do know."[141] By contrast, we neither know nor perceive
the possibility and the reality of God and immortality, since they are
not conditions of the moral law but merely conditions of the highest
good, which is the necessary object of a free will. In the second
place, the idea of freedom is the only one of the ideas of pure reason
which can be classified among the *res facti*. It is "the only concept of
the supersensible which . . . proves its objective reality in nature."[142]
It is "the only one [*das einzige*] . . . whose object is a thing of fact
[*Thatsache*] and [must] be reckoned under the *scibilia*."[143] In this it is
distinguished from the ideas of God and immortality, which, together with the highest good (of which they are necessary condi-

tions), are objects of faith (*res Fidei, credibilia*). We should note how paragraph 91 of the third *Critique* clarifies the notion of freedom set out in the second *Critique* by indicating the distinction we must make between that freedom which is presented in the Analytic as the object of a practical knowledge and that which is affirmed in the Dialectic, under the denomination *postulate,* as the object of a rational faith.

Remarkably, the two privileges we have mentioned engender a third, which is hardly the least significant since it is because of it that freedom deserves to be considered as the linchpin of the entire critical system. "*Through the concept of freedom,* the ideas of God and immortality gain objective reality and legitimacy [*Befugniss*]." [144] Evidently this privilege decisively sanctions the priority of freedom over the other ideas. Following the proof of the objective reality of freedom, we penetrated the intelligible world and glimpsed the possibility of further knowledge of the supersensible order. Moreover, it must not be the case that freedom, having opened the door to the intelligible world, would close it on itself. Thus the hope of penetrating further into the supersensible, which remains forbidden to speculative knowledge, is not at all misguided. Thanks to the "great fruitfulness [*Fruchtbarkeit*]" of the concept of freedom, [145] we can, "in accordance with the wish of metaphysics, . . . pass beyond the limits of all possible experience," [146] and initiate with Kant a metaphysics according to ethics by restoring the theoretically unacceptable data of metaphysics (God and immortality) along practical lines. "It is, properly speaking, *only* the concept of freedom, among all the ideas of pure speculative reason, which brings [knowledge] such a great extension in the field of the super-sensuous, though it is only practical knowledge which is enlarged." [147]

We already know how this practical extension of pure reason is carried out: the moral law directs us to realize the highest good. "It is a priori (morally) necessary to bring forth the highest good through the freedom of the will." [148] The highest good must therefore be possible, and the conditions which make it possible must be granted. It will be noted that the deduction of God and immortality is not accomplished directly from the moral law but only with the intervention of freedom. This point deserves to be emphasized. "All other concepts (those of God and immortality) which, as mere ideas, are unsupported by anything in speculative reason now attach themselves to the concept of freedom and gain, *with it and through it*, stability and objective reality. That is, their possibility is proved by the fact that there really is freedom, for this idea is revealed by the moral law." [149] Freedom acquires its status from the fact that it is manifest in us through the moral law (freedom is a *factum rationis*) and in the world through effective acts (freedom is a *res facti*). On one hand, it must not be forgotten that the moral law emanates from freedom and that as a result it is freedom which, through the practical law, "supplies material for cognition of other supersensibles (the moral final purpose and the conditions of its attainability)." [150] The idea of freedom "is revealed by the moral law." [151] Then, too, the moral law leads directly to the concept of freedom. By contrast, we have no direct consciousness of God and immortality. We experience our freedom, and it is our freedom of which we are conscious. Freedom is inside us, and it is in part this inwardness which accounts for its fruitfulness. "The supersensible within us" [152] (freedom) enables us to determine "the supersensible without us," [153] that is, "the supersensible *above* us" (God) and "the supersensible *after* us" (immortality). [154] "Only the concept of freedom enables us to find the unconditioned for the conditioned and the intelligible for the sensuous *without going outside ourselves.*" [155] But, on the other hand, the inwardness of freedom is not without a component of exteriority, for freedom is necessarily revealed in nature. Freedom "is meant to actualize in the world of sense the purpose proposed by its laws," that is, "the highest good." [156] Or, at the very least, it must exert itself to succeed in this aim as far as possible. The full realization of the highest good would be impossible, however, if we did not admit God and immortality "as the conditions under which alone we . . . can conceive the possibility of that *effect* of the use of our freedom in conformity with law." [157] But correlatively, it is only because freedom "establishes its reality in actions as a fact" [158] that we can, at the practical level, deduce God and immortality.

The determination of both [concepts], God and the soul (in respect of its immortality) alike, can only take place by means of predicates which, although they are only possible from a supersensible ground, must yet prove their reality *in experience,* for *thus alone* can they make possible a cognition of a quite supersensible Being. The only concept [*der einzige Begriff*] of this kind to be met with in human reason is that of the freedom of men under moral laws, along with the final purpose which reason prescribes by these laws. Of these two [the moral laws and the final purpose], the first are useful for ascribing to the author of nature, the second for ascribing to man, those properties [*Eigenschaften*] which contain the necessary condition of the possibility of both [God and the soul], so that from this idea we can conclude as to the existence and constitution [*Beschaffenheit*] of these beings *which are otherwise quite hidden from us.*[159]

The idea of freedom, which is immediately determined by the moral law, mediates the determination of the two other ideas of reason. Hence the affirmation of God and immortality cannot claim the same degree of certainty as freedom. Indeed, some of Kant's more curious formulations might lead us to think that, strictly speaking, only the idea of freedom is invested with objective reality. "Of all intelligible objects absolutely [*schlechterdings*] *nothing* [is known] except freedom (through the moral law), and even this only in so far as it is a presupposition inseparable from the moral law."[160] "One cannot provide or prove objective reality for *any idea but for the idea of freedom* [my emphasis]; and this is the case because freedom is the condition of the *moral law,* whose reality is an axiom."[161] The privileged place Kant grants the idea of freedom can be explained by the fact that the ideas of God and immortality are granted as postulates and for that very reason are the object of a lesser degree of certainty.

Notwithstanding the place of privilege which freedom enjoys among the ideas of pure reason, it remains mysterious in many respects. It is incomprehensible (*unbegreiflich*) and impenetrable (*unerforschlich*).[162] It is "the transcendental predicate of the causality of a being which belongs to the world of sense."[163] It does not itself belong to the sensuous. It is an "incomprehensible character [*unbegreifliche Eigenschaft*]"[164] whose ground is "inscrutable"[165] and whose nature escapes our intelligence.

Granted, we have a certain practical understanding of freedom, insofar as we know beyond all doubt that freedom is the condition of the moral law, which we do know. But this practical understanding extends no further than this. We know *that* we are free, but we do not know what our freedom is in itself. "Hence we understand perfectly well what freedom is, practically (when it is a question of duty), whereas we cannot without contradiction even think of wishing to understand theoretically the causality of freedom (or its nature)."[166] If we knew the nature of freedom, we could thereby claim access to direct knowledge of the free being as such. But we do not have such knowledge. The actual nature of a free being remains beyond the limits of our knowledge, for we cannot know "what the object may be to which this kind of causality is attributed." [167]

Freedom in itself is not merely unknowable, it is also unexplainable. The knowledge of freedom remains limited precisely because the objective reality of the concept "can in no way be shown according to natural laws or in any possible experience." [168] For all possible explanation ends where determination by natural laws ends. We can and must admit *that* freedom is possible, but we cannot explain *in what way* it is possible. [169] Indeed, we know in what way the practical objective reality of freedom is established: it is through the mediation of the moral law. But the consciousness of the moral law is a fact of reason which simply imposes itself without thus explaining anything further. [170] Similarly, we know in what way a categorical imperative is possible: its possibility depends on the necessary presupposition of the idea of freedom. "But how this presupposition itself is possible can never be discerned by any human reason." [171] Only by transforming freedom into nature would we be able to explain how free causality is possible. Thus, those who consider freedom a psychological property, who think to explain it as a natural faculty by a close examination of the nature of the soul, undermine both freedom and the moral law. To be able to explain freedom, we would have to understand how free intelligible causality produces its sensible effects. Even if we could identify the empirical effects which reveal freedom, we would nevertheless be unable to understand the relation between the intelligible cause and the sensible effect, since "experience can exemplify the relation of cause to effect only as subsisting between two objects of experience." [172] Freedom can be counted among the *scibilia* because it produces actions in experience, yet it remains incomprehensible since it is not itself an object of experience. Freedom is revealed *in* the world, although it is not *of* the world.

The preceding analyses enable us to show the fundamental place autonomy of the will occupies in Kant's practical philosophy. Considered first as a logical implication of the categorical imperative, the principle of autonomy then appeared as the key to the explanation of that imperative, and then as the power which synthesizes the will of the finite rational being and the universal law. Consequently, the fact that the existence of the moral law was given by a fact of reason

gave us sufficient grounds to affirm the existence of its real condition. In this way the objective reality of freedom was solidly established. Freedom is the *ratio essendi* of the moral law, which in turn is
the *ratio cognoscendi* of freedom.

It is important not to interrupt the movement of Kant's thought
but to work through his manifold analysis before reflecting on the
notion of autonomy itself and attempting—within the limits imposed on us by our own finitude—any insight into the essence of
freedom.[173] We must admit that the several paths we have followed
with Kant have left some crucial problems unresolved, and these we
must consider now. In the first place, we will turn our reflection to
the very notion of moral autonomy, a notion "so much the richer
and more fruitful"[174] that it remains shrouded in an as yet un-
thematized and unanalyzed obscurity. In the second place, we will
endeavor to determine how those other features which accompany
the freedom of a finite rational being can be articulated according to
the highest form of freedom, that is, autonomy.

Autonomy of the Will

What does moral autonomy consist in? Posing the question in these
terms already orients our answer and circumscribes the subject of
our reflection. For in a certain sense, all willing (as all practical reason) is autonomous, even when, under the attraction of sensuous
impulses, it adopts an empirically conditioned principle as the subjective principle of its action. The will which chooses the principle of
happiness as the maxim of its action acts in virtue of a principle
posed by the will itself. In autonomously choosing such a maxim, it
actually chooses to be heteronomous. Even the immoral will is always rational, and "in any way good,"[175] in view of the end it pur-
sues, but its autonomy gives way in exhaustion to heteronomy. As
Guerolt remarks:

If the principle which reason chooses is itself not rational, but sensible,
with respect to its content, then reason is indistinguishable from the inclination to which it is subordinated in the moment of decision. It becomes
the instrument of sensibility: an absurdity for reason and a perversion for
the will. For that which is independent now autonomously determines
itself by placing itself in a state of dependence. What is unconditioned is
made to be conditioned. What is an end in itself becomes a mere instrument, and transforms desires, or their objects, into ends in themselves.[176]

Thus heteronomy always implies a certain autonomy. But this autonomy is merely *formulaic,* for when reason adopts a principle arising from sensibility, it is only autonomous in form. By contrast, when the principle of action is rational both because reason adopts it and because it arises from reason itself, autonomy obtains both in the formula and materially. This is moral autonomy. The law which the autonomous rational being posits is nothing other than the moral law, that is, the law of *its* will.[177] It is in this precise and narrow sense that Kant uses the term autonomy.

In a finite rational being, moral autonomy presents two complementary and inseparable aspects. As rational, the human being establishes for itself the moral law which is imposed on every being endowed with reason. But as finite, the human being must impose on itself obedience to this law, which now takes the form of an imperative. Without risk of contradiction we can affirm that we both *are* autonomous and *ought to be* autonomous, since (at least in a being which cannot pretend to holiness) obedience to the law does not necessarily accompany the mere enunciation of that law by autonomous reason. Only a rational being can be autonomous, yet the human being is not only rational. Hence, for us autonomy is at once the ground and the principle of our obligation. Our autonomy places us under obligation and, at the same time, it is our autonomy to which we are obliged. We will analyze these two aspects of autonomy in turn.

It is not easy to specify what autonomy consists in. We would do well to recall that even though the concept of autonomy constitutes the central point of his entire practical philosophy, Kant never sets it out thematically. Moreover, his many formulations are ambiguous, and they give rise to opposing interpretations. Heidegger, for instance, took autonomy to be the outline of the moral law, which "reason as free *gives* to itself."[178] On the other hand, G. Krüger, in express opposition to Heidegger, maintains that the moral law is a given (*donné*) rather than a human construct.[179] Both of these interpretations find support in certain passages, and indeed it would be difficult to draw the debate to a close. Instead we prefer to rephrase the question and ask if these are not perhaps complementary postures with respect to Kant's thought. Perhaps it is not a matter of inquiring whether for Kant the law is a given *or* a law which we give ourselves, since the alternatives do not necessarily force themselves

or us as an opposition. Rather it is a matter of examining whether it
is possible to maintain without contradiction that the moral law is
both a fact and a construct.

At the end of the second *Critique,* Kant writes, "Two things fill the
mind with every new and increasing admiration and awe, the oftener
and more steadily we reflect on them: the starry heavens above me
and the moral law within me. I do not merely conjecture them and
seek them as though obscured in darkness or in the transcendent
region beyond my horizon: I see them before me, and I associate
them directly with the consciousness of my own existence."[180] The
moral law is in us. We discover it in us without having to search
it out, for it arises from the very structure of our being, insofar as
we are rational beings. "Were it not given us from within [*in uns
gegeben*], we should never by an ratiocination subtilize it into existence or win over our will to it."[181] Reason does not produce the law,
yet it knows it, and indeed this knowledge is twofold (*une co-
naissance*), since reason, by revealing the law, also reveals itself. As we
have seen, the fact of reason is as much the fact of the existence of
reason in us as the fact of the existence of the moral law in us. To
deny the presence of the law would be to deny the presence of reason. The principle of morality is "*in the reason of all men and embodied* [*einverleibt*] in their being."[182] The moral law is not inherent in
human nature but rather in the nature of reason itself and thus, as a
result, in human nature, to the extent that it is endowed with reason.
The law is coextensive with reason. It is not merely the lot of human
beings, however, since by right it belongs to all rational beings, in-
cluding "the Infinite Being as the supreme intelligence."[183] The autonomous will is "the pure will," that is, the will of the rational qua
rational, the human will to the extent that it is, in essence, purely
rational. The autonomous will is just pure practical reason. Freedom
is reason. Reason, which conceives freedom, recognizes itself in it.
The concept of freedom is reason's mirror.

Although the moral law is for us a given, in the sense that it is
found in our reason, it does not impose itself on us in the same way
that the laws of physics govern the physical body. Every stone which
falls is subject to the law of falling bodies, but the stone does not
represent that law to itself. Only a rational being can act according to
the representation it makes of the laws or principles which orient its
action. "Everything in nature works according to laws. Only a ra-

tional being has the capacity of acting according to the conception of laws, i.e., according to principles."[184] The human being is conscious of the principles according to which it determines itself. But among these principles, the principle of morality occupies a unique and privileged place, since all others must be subordinated to it. Hence, the consciousness of the moral law has an original and irreplaceable significance. Whereas I may be conscious of certain desires or inclinations affecting my sensibility without thereby judging that I ought to permit them to guide my conduct, I cannot be conscious of the moral law without by that very fact recognizing it as obligatory for me. "Through reason we are *conscious* of a law to which all our maxims are subject."[185] I know the moral law through reason. Through reason, too, "I recognize myself as existing in a universal and necessary . . . connection" with the intelligible world.[186] I recognize the moral law as the law of *my* will. I appropriate it. I approve it (though this does not mean that I obey it out of necessity). The recognition of a law discovered in oneself is freedom—a freedom belonging inalienably to everyone, "even the most malicious villain," since "he acknowledges the authority of this law even while transgressing it."[187] Moreover, the consciousness of the moral law makes us conscious of ourselves as members of the intelligible world. "For it is our reason itself which through the supreme and unconditioned practical law recognizes itself . . . as belonging to the pure world of the understanding."[188]

Because it freely assumes the weight of the law which it bears in itself, reason is rightly considered the author of the law. If reason does not strictly speaking *create* the law, since the law is given as a fact, it *decrees* the law and establishes it as the highest end which can be imposed on every being endowed with reason. For Kant says, "It does not necessarily follow that the law-giver is the author of the law."[189] The law appears as both a given and a construct. And it would misconstrue Kant's thought to emphasize either of these two aspects at the expense of the other. He himself considered them indissolubly united. "In order to regard this law without any misinterpretation as given [*als gegeben*], one must note that it is . . . the sole fact of pure reason, which by it proclaims itself as *originating law* [*als ursprünglich gesetzgebend*]."[190] "This legislation, however, must *be found* [*angetroffen*] in every rational being. It must be able to *arise* [*entspringen*] from his will."[191] Kant employs numerous formulas to remind us that reason is the faculty which establishes the moral law: The human being is "subject to . . . pure practical laws given by its own reason." [192] "Pure reason is practical of itself alone, and it *gives* [my emphasis] (to man) a universal law, which we call the *moral law*." [193] Moreover, insofar as reason is not a faculty outside of us but an essential attribute of our nature, it is appropriate to specify that the human being, far from receiving the moral law passively, can be rightly considered the originator of the law. Thus, since it is conscious of itself as a thing-in-itself, the human being "views his existence . . . as determinable only by laws which *he gives* to himself through reason [*es sich durch Vernunft selbst gibt*]." [194] Properly understood, this amounts to one of the two standpoints [195] from which man can consider himself: as a noumenon he "gives to himself [*sich selbst gibt*]" [196] a moral legislation to which he is subject.

The course we have followed in the preceding analysis was intended to make us recognize that the human being is the only author of the moral legislation it must obey. This claim receives its fundamental significance when we specify that the human being is only obliged to obey the moral law because he is its author. Autonomy is the ground of obligation, since apart from autonomy there would be no moral law at all. Only that law which the subject poses itself can be absolutely unconditioned, thus guaranteeing the strictly disinterested character of moral action. Only the law of *its* will can be a moral law. [197] Hence the subject is obliged to obey the law only insofar as it arises from its own will. "The will is thus not only subject to the law but subject in such a way that it must be regarded also as self-legislative and only for this reason as being subject to the law (of which it can regard itself as the author)." [198] If the human being participates in the sublime at all, it is only because he is subject to the moral law "in so far as he is *legislative* with reference to the law and *subject to it only for this reason*." [199]

Certainly the legislative act is not left to the caprice (*arbitraire*) of the subject. The positing of the law is no less unconditioned than the law itself, for a free will cannot act without the law. It posits the law in a manner which is at once free and necessary, but it is just because it is free that it necessarily gives itself as a law the universal form of all law. [200] It is true that the will does not choose from among several alternative legislations. But this in no way diminishes the freedom of the act which institutes the law. If we took freedom to mean mere freedom of choice, we would have to acknowledge that "only choice can be called free" and that "the [legislative] will cannot be called either free or unfree." [201] But in fact, choice does not constitute freedom. It merely expresses a certain form of freedom—one which, as we shall see, is hardly the highest form. In the legislative act, on the other hand, freedom and necessity coincide: the legislative will is free precisely in that it promulgates the law through the necessity of its own nature. In laying down that pure law which constitutes it as rational, the will itself is established. It is even "incapable of constraint." [202]

Therefore, autonomy constitutes the very morality of the moral law. From Kant's perspective, it is no exaggeration to claim that no moral law imposed by an external authority could ever even deserve the name "moral law." We could even ask whether such a law was not simply immoral. In any case, Kant objects vigorously to every theological morality. It would be the ruin of morality itself to base it on a divinely imposed, external injunction: a system of morals grounded on the concept of a divine will "would be directly *opposed to morality.*" [203] Kant is not content merely with the assertion that it is "not to be understood that the assumption of the existence of God is necessary as a ground of all obligation in general." [204] He wants to claim in addition that we must not even admit such a ground. We must never think that an alternative ground of morality would be acceptable, supposing autonomy had been refused to man, or that the divine will had made up for the loss of autonomy by imposing an allegedly moral law on rational beings. The ground of all obligation "rests . . . *solely* on the autonomy of reason itself." [205] Let us make no mistake: the exclusivity, or the "monopoly" which autonomy enjoys, does not constitute a merely *factual* privilege; it is a privilege *of right*. Without autonomy there is no morality. The authority of the moral law does not *and cannot* flow from the divine will. It cannot flow from the divine will because—by right and by necessity—its only source must be the autonomy of practical reason. It cannot flow from the divine will because—in fact—our theoretical reason is incapable of proving the existence of God. Under the circumstances, the fact guarantees the right. The domain of speculative reason had to be limited in order to guarantee the autonomy of practical reason. Moral action becomes possible through the limitation of our knowledge. If we could prove the existence of God, "most actions con-

forming to the law would be done from fear, few would be done
from hope, none from duty."²⁰⁶ The finitude of the mind conditions
the eminent dignity of our moral nature, and this reveals once again
the harmony of speculative and practical reason.

"In [human beings], the law has the form of an imperative. For
though we can suppose that men as rational beings have a pure will,
since they are affected by wants and sensuous motives we cannot
suppose them to have a holy will, a will incapable of any maxims
which conflict with the moral law."²⁰⁷ The will of the human, as a
rational being, is a pure will, an *objective* will which imposes its own
law on itself as the principle of its action. But the human will, insofar
as it is also subject to sensuous motives according to its *subjective*
constitution, does not conform itself perfectly to reason, nor is it
necessarily determined by the moral law. The moral law is holy;
human will is not. Hence, the relation of such a will to the law "is
one of dependence [*Abhängigkeit*] under the name of 'obligation'
[*Verbindlichkeit*] . . . [which] implies a constraint [*Nötigung*]."²⁰⁸ This
will is thus both spontaneous and receptive, legislator and subject.
Its "subjection to the law" reveals its "subjective imperfection."²⁰⁹
As Heidegger observes, "Finite reason is receptive even in its spontaneity."²¹⁰ This receptivity is revealed in me in the form of a feeling
of respect for the law. "The consciousness of a free submission
[*Unterwerfung*] of the will to the law, combined with an inevitable
constraint [*Zwang*] imposed only by our own reason on all inclinations, is respect for the law."²¹¹

In a finite rational being, the positing of the unconditioned law is
absolutely necessary and ineluctable. But obedience to the law remains contingent. In other words, the will's free imposition of the
law on itself does not entail its free submission to the law. The contingency of moral action indicates that the human being has the
power of opposing itself to the law, as well as the power of imposing
the law on itself. Moral experience, in addition to revealing the autonomy of the will, makes us aware that we are free either to conform or not to conform to the law.²¹² Thus two forms of freedom
coexist in us: moral autonomy and free choice. Whereas the pure
legislative will (*Wille*) lays down the moral law as the formal principle
for the determination of action, the human will (*Wille*)—the rational will affected by sensibility—stands "halfway between its a
priori principle which is formal and its a posteriori incentive which

is material."²¹³ It is as though at a "crossroads."²¹⁴ Thus it appears to
be endowed with a power of free choice (*Willkür*). For our "choice is
sensibly affected and therefore does not of itself conform with the
pure will but often opposes it."²¹⁵

Now we must orient our reflection towards an examination of
this *Willkür*. Nevertheless, before we undertake this analysis, it will
be useful to underscore one point in particular: is it not remarkable
that, precisely because the concept of freedom comprises two different forms of freedom, the idea of autonomy itself divides into two
notions closely linked to one another, yet distinct? Insofar as it is
legislative, the human will is autonomous; insofar as it is not necessarily determined by the law, it receives the principle of autonomy as
a categorical imperative. Two paths open up to the will. When it
determines itself solely with respect to the form of the universal law,
the will chooses to follow "its" own course, and by doing so, to affirm its freedom, that is, its "*independence* of everything except the
moral law."²¹⁶ On the other hand, when the will determines itself
with respect to an empirical principle, a heteronomy of its free
choice arises, that is, "a *dependence* on natural laws in following some
impulse or inclination."²¹⁷

It is the strange fate of a being which both *is* and nevertheless
must *make* itself free that the autonomy of its will is not merely a
given (*donné*) but also a task (*ordonné*). Employing a contemporary
vocabulary, we could speak of factual and authentic autonomy. Nor
would it be unfaithful to Kant's thought to claim that the celebrated
maxim, Become what you are! imposes itself on the autonomous will
of the rational being. The human will must in effect reclaim the autonomy which it, insofar as it is in essence rational, possesses from all
eternity. This is the paradoxical situation of a will which is alienated
from itself by the disruptions of sensibility. The human will must be
what it already, as a pure will, is. Thus, there exists within the human
being a division between the objective, intelligible will and the subjective will affected by sensibility. The categorical imperative reveals
this division²¹⁸ and requires (*ordonne*) that it be overcome. The moral
law which the autonomous will posits "commands neither more nor
less than this very autonomy."²¹⁹ Put another way, freedom takes
itself for its object and aims at its own realization. "The will," Hegel
will say, "is the free will which wills the free will."²²⁰

It is this noncoincidence of man with himself which brings about the disjunction within the notion of autonomy. But the disjunction itself is evidently only the correlate of that double standpoint according to which man can be considered a member of the intelligible world and of the sensible world at one and the same time. The noumenal man *is* autonomous and law-giving because he imposes on the rational and sensible man a law which he must obey if he wants to *become* autonomous. "Man as subject of moral legislation proceeding from the concept of freedom, in which he is subject to a law he gives to himself (*homo noumenon*), is to be regarded as different from the sensible man endowed with reason (*specie diversus*); but different only from a practical point of view."[221]

Precisely because the will is autonomous, the obligation to become autonomous which it imposes on itself can exercise a constraint which is not incompatible with freedom of the will. For it is quite autonomously that I prescribe for myself the duty of autonomy. The constraint which inheres in duty springs from my own free will; it concerns a "self-constraint" in no way prejudicial to freedom.[222] Rousseau rightly affirms that "obedience to the law one has prescribed for oneself is freedom."[223]

The human will ought to be autonomous. It must follow, therefore, that it can be autonomous. If freedom is a duty, the duty implies freedom. The imperative of autonomy would be absurd if the will could not be determined by pure practical reason alone and thus reassert its independence with respect to natural laws and sensuous motives. Our will is admittedly not an "absolutely good will,"[224] since it can take a maxim contrary to the moral law as the principle of its action. But it is nevertheless "a possible will which is absolutely good,"[225] because it is capable of determining itself by the moral law alone. Considered in this light, autonomy no longer appears as a fact of reason but as an ideal to be pursued. "Our own will, so far as it would act only under the condition of a universal legislation rendered possible by its maxims—this will ideally possible for us is the proper object of respect."[226]

Kant says in the *Grundlegung* that "a free will and a will under moral laws are identical."[227] This assertion is unquestionably ambiguous, yet its very ambiguity is also the source of its richness. To extract the deepest significance of this formula, we can consider it at two levels of interpretation, corresponding to the two aspects we have distinguished in the notion of autonomy.

First of all, we could consider the will free *when* it obeys the moral law. Did Kant then want to maintain that only that will is free which acts from duty? But if this were the case, would we not have to admit that the bad will is not free at all? This would amount to a denial of evil, since an action cannot be qualified morally unless it proceeds from freedom. Such an interpretation cannot withstand careful examination, especially when we place it in the context of a system which recognizes not only the reality of moral evil but also the possibility of regeneration. Evidently we must seek out a more supple and less restrictive interpretation. Obedience to the moral law reinstates the will's freedom. It answers to a demand which arises from the will itself, namely, the demand to become autonomous. The will realizes its freedom in full only when it submits to the principle of morality. Obedience to the law is freedom. Yet for a will which is not infallibly determined by the law, obedience always remains contingent. Full freedom is inaccessible to us precisely because our will will never follow the law out of necessity. In one who is holy, freedom merges with necessity, whereas the virtuous being must always strive to reduce the contingency of moral actions as much as possible and thus to make them more necessary. This possibility of progress towards holiness seems to authorize the claim that there are degrees of freedom. A person "proves his freedom in the highest degree by the very fact that he cannot oppose the voice of duty." [228] The human being is thus freer the more completely it submits to the moral law. In Heidegger's words: "By submitting to the law, I submit myself to myself *qua* pure reason. In submitting to myself, I raise myself to myself as a free being capable of self-determination." [229]

The identification of the free will with the will subjected to moral laws can be interpreted in another way, which does not oppose the foregoing but instead completes and even confirms it. We could consider the will free *because* it gives the law and is thus subject to a law which it institutes itself (see pp. 75–76). [230] Being subject (*unterworfen*), or subordinated (*untergeordnet*) to the moral law means recognizing it, not necessarily obeying it. Kant establishes a clear distinction between a will which is *subject* to moral laws (*unter moralischen Gesetzen*) and one which *obeys* moral laws. [231] Whether good or bad, this human will is always subject to the law. Someone who commits a wrong does not cease to be a lawgiver by doing so. "He acknowledges [*er erkennt*] the authority of this law even while transgressing it."[232] He acknowledges the validity of the categorical imperative,[233] and he experiences an inward resistance even while violating it.[234] The recognition of the moral law is freedom. In this sense the will of the finite rational being is always free. Autonomy of the will is not only the supreme form of freedom, it is the original and essential freedom "which lies at the foundation of all moral laws and accountability to them."[235] The autonomous will makes the human being a responsible being endowed with free choice. "Man *himself* must make or have made himself into whatever, in a moral sense, whether good or evil, he is or is to become. Either condition must be an effect of his free choice [*Willkür*]; for otherwise he could not be held responsible for it and could therefore be *morally* neither good nor evil."[236]

5   The Self-Negation of Freedom: Radical Evil

Intelligible Free Will

In man autonomy of the will is not only a given but also the object of a choice. Precisely because the human being is capable of choosing a maxim which either conforms to or opposes the moral law, autonomy represents an ideal to be pursued. Great caution must be exercised not to confuse the two forms of freedom which coexist in us (see pp. 78–79). The act by which the pure will lays down the universal moral law is different from the act by which the will conforms to the law or transgresses it.[1] Just how these two acts of the will are to be articulated constitutes the crux of Kant's problematic in the practical realm. Yet interestingly, this central problem, which, without question, always occupied Kant's attention, seems to have acquired its full importance and acuity only gradually, as he elaborated his practical philosophy. It cannot escape our notice that from the *Grundlegung* (1785) to *Religion Within the Limits of Reason Alone* (1793), Kant's reflection describes a trajectory which leads us from the analysis of the legislative will (*Wille*) to examination of the fundamental choice made by the free will (*Willkür*). At the midpoint of that trajectory, the second *Critique* initiates the discussion by concluding the analysis of the autonomous will, which had already been investigated in the *Grundlegung,* and outlining the analysis of free choice, which would be completed later in *Religion within the Limits of Reason Alone.* Although the problem pervades each of these works, the tone differs, depending on which of the two notions is emphasized. In the second *Critique,* for example, Kant finds it necessary to place moral autonomy in the foreground (in the first chapter of the Analytic) without, however, neglecting the notion of free choice (which he treats in part in the Critical Elucidation of the Analytic of Pure Practical Reason). It seems as if the two ideas cannot be analyzed together without one or the other attempting, at the expense of the other, to monopolize the entire reflection. This is enormously

important for the interpretation of Kant's thought: the problem of
the relation and coexistence in one being of a law-giving will side by
side with free choice appears so difficult to articulate and resolve
within the framework of his philosophy that Kant himself seems
never to have addressed it directly. His thought on the subject un-
folds in a variety of strategies relatively unrelated to one another.[2]
Hence the confrontation between *Wille* and *Willkür* transpires only
intermittently, and our interpretation must glean some way of resolving the problem from hints scattered here and there.

The fact that Kant's terminology establishes a progressively
clearer distinction between the legislative will (*Wille*) and free choice
(*Willkür*) testifies to the increasing interest he invests in the problem.
But significantly, we must wait for *The Metaphysics of Morals* to see
Kant take note of this evolution and attempt finally to specify the
meaning of the two terms, thereby making explicit a vocabulary
which until then had been variable and indecisive.[3] "Laws proceed
from the will; maxims from choice [*Von dem Willen gehen die Gesetze
aus; von der Willkür die Maximen*]."[4] It is not necessary, as the language
employed might easily suggest, to distinguish two different faculties
in us, will (*volonté*) and free choice (*libre arbitre*), nor even to speak of
two sorts of will.[5] The point is merely not to confuse two complementary aspects of the will, according to which it is considered as a
legislative will or as an elective will.[6]

Wille and *Willkür* are both linked to the faculty of desire, defined
by Kant as "the faculty [in a being] . . . of causing, through its ideas,
the reality of the objects of these ideas."[7] This capacity is coextensive
with life itself and does not characterize the human as such, since it
can be found also in the animal. It becomes specifically human only
when liking (*bon gré; das Belieben*) intervenes, as the two definitions
Kant provides attest:

> The faculty of desiring according to concepts is called *the faculty of
> doing or forbearing as one pleases* [*nach Belieben*] insofar as the ground deter-
> mining it to action is found in the faculty of desire itself and not in the
> object. Insofar as it is combined with the consciousness of the capacity
> of its action to produce its object, it is called choice [*Willkür*]; if not so
> combined, its act is called a wish [*Wunsch*].[8]

> The faculty of desire whose internal ground of determination and,
> consequently, even whose liking [*das Belieben*] is found in the reason of the
> subject is called the will [*Wille*].[9]

Yet clearly the term *Belieben,* as employed in these two different contexts, does not encompass the same reality in each case. Applied to *Willkür,* it designates the aspect of contingency which belongs to the action of a being which can either act or refrain from acting and can adopt any given rule of action in preference over another. By contrast, when applied to *Wille, Belieben* indicates the free necessity with which the autonomous will, which is "incapable of constraint,"[10] gives birth to the moral law (see pp. 76–77). The law which the *Wille* decrees serves as the principle for the determination of the *Willkür. Wille* and *Willkür* are two aspects of the will which differ from each other as the legislative power differs from the executive.[11] "The will is the faculty of desire regarded not (like choice) in relation to action, but rather as the ground determining choice to action."[12]

Now we must turn our attention to the notion of free choice itself. We begin by examining what the freedom of free choice consists in, and then we consider the use free choice makes of that freedom. Kant often characterizes the freedom proper to free choice in formulas which assume the aspect of definitions; but these are spread throughout his work so that, here again, it is the task of interpretation to reveal, or even to introduce, a logical order among the key passages in order to illuminate Kant's thought.

The notion of a maxim, which occupies a central position in every analysis of *Willkür,* provides a preliminary characterization of the freedom of free choice. This is evident in the famous formula from *The Metaphysics of Morals,* "Maxims [proceed] from choice."[13] Moreover, this formula follows a line which Kant had already maintained when he defined the will as the faculty of acting according to rules and maxims. A maxim is a "subjective principle of acting,"[14] which the rational subject adopts and following which he proposes to act. The maxim expresses the subject's disposition. It indicates how he intends to act. "The rule which the agent adopts on subjective grounds as his principle is called his maxim."[15] Just as the freedom of the autonomous will consists in the establishment of the objective law, the freedom of free choice is characterized primarily by the faculty of adopting subjective rules of action and acting only in view of these rules.[16] This faculty, in effect, guarantees the independence of the human will with regard to every object which might influence it.[17] "*Good* or *evil* always indicates a relation to the will so far as it is determined by the law of reason to make something its object, for the will is never determined directly by the object and our conception of it; rather the will is a faculty which can make an object real."[18] This faculty enables the will to distance itself from the object. The maxim plays a mediating role: in order for an object to become an incentive, that is, "a subjective determining ground of a will,"[19] the incentive must have been admitted beforehand in the rule of action of the will. Ultimately, it is always the maxim which determines the action and the will which determines itself to act. The freedom of free choice "is of a wholly unique nature in that an incentive [*Triebfeder*] can determine [free choice] [*Willkür*] to an action *only so far as the individual has incorporated it into his maxim* (has made it the general rule in accordance with which he will conduct himself)."[20] In other words, no incentive is determinative in itself. The human being, by a free act, confers a determinative power on a particular incentive. Hence, the absolute spontaneity of free choice is never fettered by the influence of any incentive. This is the most elementary aspect of human freedom, the basis of all moral culture and all education in freedom. "We must see," says Kant, "that the child should accustom himself to act in accordance with 'maxims,' and not from certain ever-changing springs of action [*Triebfedern*]."[21]

The first consequence of the foregoing may initially seem paradoxical. Evidently we can affirm that, where we might be tempted to see only pure determinism at the level of sensuous motives, the will already exercises its power of free choice. For the will (*Willkür*) is the faculty of choosing from among sensuous motives those which will be incorporated in its maxim.[22] This means that when the will delivers itself over to heteronomy (see p. 79), it has the freedom to fix for itself the modality of its own heteronomy. If I decide in a given circumstance to act out of pity or jealousy, rather than out of duty, it is up to me to accept one or another of these motives in the maxim of my act. Already at this level it is permissible to disclose a fundamental difference between animal choice (*arbitrium brutum*) and free human choice. Whereas the animal's choice is strictly determined through the impulse which exercises the strongest hold over its sensibility, human choice is never determined, but merely influenced, by sensuous motives. It is only determined in view of the strongest incentive after having determined for itself which will be the strongest incentive.[23] The maxim is a rule no less rational for being subjective; and where there is reason, there is also freedom.

While it is not incorrect to consider the human's free choice as manifesting its freedom when it is simply choosing among sensuous motives, we must acknowledge that this is only a secondary aspect of freedom, which Kant never emphasizes and which we merely extract from the overall context of his philosophy. Doubtless it is not between sensuous motives but between sensibility and reason, between sensuous motives and the moral law—ultimately, that is, between heteronomy and autonomy—that the most fundamental choice is made. Such a choice is possible only because the human will is merely affected by sensibility, without ever being controlled by it. Sensible impulses, desires, and inclinations may well influence a free choice, but their influence will never be absolutely determinative, for between incentives and the determination to action the free choice of a maxim is always interposed. The will can therefore determine itself to act in a purely rational manner, without admitting the least sensuous incentive into its maxim. Does this mean that it may also act without incentive? Certainly not, yet the incentive which it does admit into its maxim is only the law of pure practical reason. "The moral law, in the judgment of reason, is in itself an incentive, and whoever makes it his maxim is *morally* good."[24] Thus, once again, the dignity of our will is revealed along with its finitude. Dignity accrues to it through its ability to disengage itself from the control of every *sensuous incentive* in order to act in view of the moral law alone. Its finitude, on the other hand, prevents it from being able to determine itself in respect of the moral law except by taking the law into its maxim under the heading of a *rational incentive*.[25] Whereas the animal's choice can *only* be determined by a sensuous incentive,[26] the human's choice "can be determined . . . through motives which are represented *only* by reason."[27] In the animal, determination by sensibility is a *necessity* imposed on it by its nature. In the human being, determination by reason is a *possibility* offered to it by its freedom. Free human choice is precisely a *free* choice (*eine freie Willkür*) because "it *can* be determined [*bestimmt werden kann*] to actions by pure will."[28] But this possibility is only explained by the independence which free choice enjoys with regard to sensibility—whence the (negative) definition of freedom given by Kant: the freedom of free choice (*die Freiheit der Willkür*) "is just that independence [*Unabhängigkeit*] from determination by sensible impulses [*Antriebe*]."[29]

When the moral law is revealed in us through the experience of an obligation, it reveals in addition the freedom of the autonomous will

which posits the law and that of the executive will which can choose
either for or against the law. The famous example by which Kant
illustrates the coming to consciousness of freedom is very significant
in this respect. A man ordered to make a false deposition against an
honorable man, under pain of death, would consider it possible to
overcome his love of life and follow the moral law. "Whether he
would or not he perhaps will not venture to say; but that it would be
possible for him he would certainly admit without hesitation (see
p. 62)."[30] Just by revealing to us that the law arises from our will,
moral experience indicates as well that we have the power of subjecting or not subjecting ourselves to the law. That the human being
has the power of following the moral law, even when such obedience
requires of him that he overcome his desire for life and resist the
terror of death, proves that free choice is in no way subject to sensuous motives, however strong or compelling they may be.[31] "This
law is the only law which informs us of the independence of our will
[Willkür] from determination by all other incentives (of our freedom) and at the same time of the accountability of all our actions."[32]
Indeed, if the moral law is the ratio cognoscendi of the freedom of free
choice, that freedom is the ratio essendi of our moral responsibility. It
is perfectly logical, as a result, that in revealing our free choice to us,
the moral law makes us conscious at the same time of the accountability of all our acts. This also explains how Kant, in joining both
forms of freedom—Wille and Willkür—in a single formula, was able
to claim that "freedom . . . lies at the foundation of all moral laws and
accountability to them. . . . Without transcendental freedom, which
is its proper meaning, and which is alone a priori practical, no moral
law and no accountability to it are possible."[33] On the other hand,
the freedom of free choice, which cannot be grasped in an intellectual intuition, is no longer a concept of experience, even though,
insofar as it is the executive faculty of the will,[34] it is revealed in
experience by its actions (see the analysis of freedom as a res facti,
pp. 63–67). Moreover, it would remain unknown to us if it were
not capable of being deduced from the moral law: "The concept of
the freedom of the will [Willkür] does not precede the consciousness
of the moral law in us but is deduced from the determinability of our
will [Willkür] by this law as an unconditional command."[35]

    "Human choice . . . can be determined to actions by a pure
will."[36] This means that in addition to conforming to the will's decree, it can also "resist" it (widerstreben).[37] The will, as Wille, wills the

law. But as *Willkür* it can also not will it. This initial discordance, this failure rooted in the very heart of the will, explains how in a finite rational being the law assumes the form of an imperative. "The categorical imperative implies on man's part an obedience and submission of his free choice to the law." [38] Free choice is subject to the law when it incorporates it in its maxim as an incentive, as the sole subjective principle of action. Only then is the voice of reason, the "heavenly voice" present in everyone, no longer stifled by external considerations which could exercise a determining influence on the heart. [39] "Where the moral law speaks [*spricht*] there is no longer, objectively, a free choice [*keine freie Wahl*] as regards what is to be done." [40] Through obedience to the law, the division which had split the human will is healed (see pp. 79–80). Henceforth *Willkür* becomes *Wille* and the law of the legislative will becomes the "law of the freely choosing will [*freien Willkür*]." [41]

In light of the foregoing analysis, we can locate the freedom of human free choice in relation to animal choice, on one hand, and in relation to the divine will, on the other. While the animal is determined by sensibility alone, the divine being is determined by reason alone. The human being, by contrast, is a sort of hybrid—at once rational and sensible. As rational, the human being is endowed with a "power of choosing its own course of conduct [*sich selbst eine Lebensweise auszuwählen*] and not being restricted to a singular course [*an eine einzige*], as other animals are." [42] As sensible, the human being possesses a will endowed with the faculty of choosing a maxim conforming to or opposing the moral principle, yet which is not thereby determined to follow only the moral law, as the will of a perfect being would be. "If reason infallibly determines the will, the actions which such a being recognizes as objectively necessary are also subjectively necessary. That is, the will is a faculty of choosing only that which [*der Wille ist ein Vermögen, nur dasjenige zu wählen, was*] reason, independently of inclination, recognizes as practically necessary, i.e., as good." [43] Because it is not restricted to a single course of conduct dictated entirely by sensibility, as the animals are, the human being is free. Nevertheless it is a finite freedom, a merely human freedom, since it is not determined uniquely by the moral law, as is the divine being. Now we must turn to this contrast between the finitude of free human choice and the fullness of the freedom of the infinite being.

While autonomy of the will represents the highest degree of freedom, free human choice is only a degraded and inferior freedom. The possibility of choosing a maxim attests to "*a limitation of the nature of the being,* in that the subjective character of its choice [*Willkür*] does not of itself agree with the objective law of practical reason." [44] The distinction between the moral law and maxims only pertains to beings in which the (imperfect) will is not determined necessarily by the representation of the good. The faculty of choosing bears witness to the finitude of human freedom. As Jean Nabert says:

> In a doctrine like Kant's, where reason and freedom are transposable, free choice (or the possibility of acting against reason and against the moral law) belongs to us insofar as we are sensible beings. There is *nothing positive* in this possibility in respect of the causality of reason. What is free in our free choice does not derive from our power to act against reason but, on the contrary, from the faculty of acting in conformity to the law. And what there is of free choice in our freedom merely testifies that the reason of a being subject to sensuous incentives may deviate from unconditioned reason. . . . The idea of choice within reason is a mark of its *weakness,* for choice indicates that the mastery of reason is not absolute. One can only make sense of it in a being which, possessing both reason and sensibility, can introduce sensuous motives into the context of its maxims. According to Kant, such is the free choice of the human, with its ability to resist reason arbitrarily." [45]

The full realization of the will's autonomy cannot eliminate the element of negativity which inheres in the very essence of human freedom. Even when free choice selects a maxim conforming to the moral law, thus reinstating its primordial freedom and fulfilling the freedom of the legislative will, the autonomy of the will nevertheless remains a merely human autonomy. For the act through which the finite being is determined in respect of the moral law is never necessary but always contingent. Although this element of negativity is not necessarily transformed into a power of negation (since free choice may yet choose the good), it remains no less true that it is the mark of our freedom's finitude. It reveals the inability of our freedom to determine itself necessarily according to the principle of morality. "Only freedom in relation to the internal legislation of reason is properly a capacity [*ein Vermögen*]; the possibility of deviating from it is an incapacity [*ein Unvermögen*]." [46]

This also clarifies the underlying meaning of Kant's formula that human choice "*can* be determined [*bestimmt werden kann*] to actions by pure will."[47] This possibility implies "independence from determination by sensible impulses (see pp. 86–87)."[48] Hence it is truly a *Vermögen* which defines the freedom of our free choice. If free choice can be determined by the pure will, however, it is not necessarily so determined: it *can* also be determined otherwise. This contrasting possibility implies, in Reinhold's phrase, "the independence of the person from the compulsion of practical reason."[49] Yet we should be cautious about taking this to represent the fundamental freedom of the human being, since the possibility of deviating from the moral law is really only an *Unvermögen*.[50]

The principle of morality, as the law of all rational beings, "is thus not limited to human beings but extends to all finite beings having reason and will; indeed, it includes the Infinite Being as the supreme intelligence."[51] God is perhaps subject to the moral law[52] but certainly not to duty. The relation of his will to the moral law is not a relation of *dependence*. The divine will suffers no compulsion: it is completely free precisely because it is determined of necessity to follow the moral law. In an infinite being, there is no way to distinguish *Wille* and *Willkür,* objective and subjective will, law and maxims. "In the supremely self-sufficing intelligence choice [*Willkür*] is correctly thought of as incapable of any maxim [*als keiner Maxime fähig*] which could not at the same time be objectively a law, and the concept of holiness, which is applied to it for this reason, elevates it not indeed above all practical laws but above all practically restrictive laws, and thus above obligation and duty."[53] Just as the possibility of deviating from the moral law expresses the weakness of human freedom, the impossibility of deviating from it reveals the supreme efficacy of the divine will. That will is completely free which *cannot* be bad, which conforms to the law of autonomy *out of necessity*. The power (*Vermögen*) of the infinite being is wholly adequate to its holy will.[54] "To reconcile the concept of freedom with the idea of God as a *necessary* Being raises no difficulty at all: for freedom consists not in the contingency [*Zufälligkeit*] of the act (that it is determined by no grounds whatever) i.e., not in indeterminism (that God must be equally capable of doing good or evil, if His actions are to be called free), but rather in absolute spontaneity."[55]

Should we consider the finite rational being equally capable of doing good or evil? In Kant's philosophy this question receives only a highly nuanced answer, which varies according to the context in which it is found. If we take the question as pertaining to a *power of opposites* in the human being, permitting it to decide in favor of the law or to resist it, it seems we must answer affirmatively. Human free choice renders obedience to the law which the autonomous will imposes contingent and makes "the actions which are recognized as objectively necessary . . . subjectively contingent." [56] Must we then conclude that the freedom of free choice consists in indeterminism? [57] Certainly not, for Kant expressly rejects the *freedom of indifference*. Granted, the human will is "undetermined," since, having the faculty of choosing, it finds itself "at the crossroads (see pp. 78–79)." [58] Yet it is always determined in respect to impulses. This means that our "disposition in respect to the moral law is never indifferent [*niemals indifferent*]." [59] How could it be, when the moral law in us is a positive incentive ($+a$)? Whoever adopts this incentive into his maxim is morally good; by contrast, one who does not choose this incentive is necessarily determined by a contrasting incentive ($-a$), and his free choice is, as a result, bad. There is no middle term: the agent is for the law or against it. If the moral law were not a positive incentive acting on free choice, evil would originate in a mere lack (*defectus, absentia*) and would merely be the result of an absence of any moral incentive. But as the law is in reality a positive principle, evil can only be the result of a real opposition between the moral law and an antagonistic incentive. Therefore it is not merely a default but a *privation,* which arises from "the destruction of the result of a positive principle." [60] And since such a destruction always requires a positive principle, evil too is positive. "Wherever there is a positive principle, and the result is Zero, there is a real opposition, that is, the principle is bound to another positive principle which negates it." [61] This shows that "a morally indifferent [*moralisch-gleichgultig*] action (*adiaphoron morale*) would be one resulting merely from natural laws, and hence standing in no relation whatsoever to the moral law" [62]— that is, in effect, quite the opposite of a free action. In this sense the freedom of indifference would be the negation of freedom. "We cannot define the freedom of free choice, in the sense of a power of acting in conformity with or in opposition to the law, for this would be a condition of totally subjective anarchy independent of every determining motive, and no action could arise from it." [63]

Thus, if we employ the expression "freedom of indifference," it is to designate the empirical free choice, which is the sensible translation of intelligible free choice. Experience attests that we have the power of choosing the subjective principle of the will from among diverse maxims.

Freedom of choice, however, cannot be defined as the capacity for making a choice to act for or against the law (*libertas indifferentiae*), as some people have tried to define it, even though choice as a phenomenon gives frequent instances of this in experience. . . . Although experience tells us that man as a sensible being exhibits a capacity to choose not only in accordance with the law but also in opposition to it, yet his freedom as an intelligible being cannot be thus defined, since appearances can never enable us to comprehend any supersensible object (such as free choice is).[64]

We cannot confuse the freedom of intelligible free choice with the empirical manifestation of that freedom. Choice expresses freedom but does not constitute it. The freedom to choose between contraries, between particular actions or objects (the freedom of indifference), leads us back to the freedom of intelligible free choice, which has the power of establishing a supreme maxim by choosing between contrary maxims. "The freedom of free choice, with regard to the choice between what conforms to and what contrasts with the law, is a respective spontaneity (*libertas phaenomenon*); in the choice of maxims of actions, it is an absolute spontaneity (*libertas noumenon*)."[65]

By broaching the subject of the choice of the supreme maxim, we arrive at a new stage in the analysis of intelligible free choice. In the foregoing considerations we intended to define, as far as we were able, the *nature* of free choice and to discern what its freedom consists in. Henceforth our reflection will focus on the *act* of this freedom itself. The choice of the supreme maxim corresponds to the act by which the human being with free choice "gives to himself" an intelligible character,[66] and thus determines the law of the causality of his will. The analysis of this act of choice raises two problems which must not be confused if we hope to clarify certain points which remain obscure in the text of *Religion Within the Limits of Reason Alone*. There Kant neglects to distinguish them and instead approaches them simultaneously, shifting his analysis back and forth from one to the other. Is it not appropriate to examine *what characterizes* this fundamental choice before considering *what is chosen?*[67]

As we know, this choice is presented under the form of an alternative: the human being must determine himself for the moral law or against it. Choosing in favor of the law means incorporating it in one's maxim as the sole incentive determining one's action. Anyone who makes such a choice is morally good; by contrast, one who chooses a contrary incentive is morally bad. Between good and evil there is no middle term whatsoever. A human cannot be partly good and partly bad. His disposition with respect to the moral law is never one of indifference. Kant's "rigorism"[68] points out one of the most distinctive characteristics of free choice: properly understood, it concerns an ethical choice, but a choice which engages our existence in its totality—a radical choice—since the act of instituting the supreme maxim determines the choice of all other secondary maxims, and thus all of our actions in the sensible world. "The disposition [*Gesinnung*], i.e., the ultimate subjective ground [*Grund*] of the adoption of maxims, can be *one* [*einzige*] only and applies universally to the *whole use* of freedom."[69]

Kant immediately specifies that this radical disposition must itself have been admitted by free choice. It is a "property of the will [*Willkür*] . . . grounded in freedom."[70] There can be no doubt that the choice of an intelligible character is a *free act,* for in ordering us to choose in its favor, the moral law clearly indicates that the choice is answerable to our free will. But it is a quite remarkable and absolutely ultimate act of freedom, for it grounds the entire use of our freedom on itself alone. The ground of good or evil can be found only "in a rule made by the will [*Willkür*] for the use of its freedom, that is, in a maxim."[71] This maxim is a "supreme maxim [*oberste Maxime*],"[72] beyond which we cannot go. It would be quite useless to inquire why the will (*Willkür*) chooses a given maxim over another, for only two possibilities are available. Either one seeks out such a ground in a "natural impulse,"[73] in which case the employment of our free choice seems to be conditioned by natural causes, which is contradictory; or one seeks out the ground "in a maxim."[74] But then one only postpones the problem, since this maxim must also have a ground, for which it would be necessary to seek out yet another maxim in such a way that we would be snared in an infinite regression.[75] Free choice freely determines the employment of its freedom, and this freedom appears to us in some way "suspended" from itself, since the ultimate subjective ground of the adoption of moral maxims remains "inscrutable to us [*uns unerforschlich*]."[76]

This ultimate subjective ground[77] of the employment of freedom cannot be deduced "from any original act of the will [*Willkür*] in time."[78] The choice of a supreme maxim is *nontemporal* for the same reason that the freedom makes it is, for that choice would not be free at all if it were subject to conditions of time. We must not think of it as a fact which could be given in experience, as if it were the first link in a series of successive conditions, but rather as an intelligible fact situated outside of every temporal series. Nevertheless, this choice must necessarily be represented as anterior to every act performed in time (though certainly this priority is merely logical, not chronological). Hence Kant defines the radical disposition as an "inborn natural constitution [*angeboren Beschaffenheit*]."[79] Good and evil are *inborn* in us "only in *this* sense, that [the particular disposition] is posited as the ground antecedent to every use of freedom in experience . . . and is thus conceived of as present in man at birth—though birth need not be the cause of it."[80] The term "inborn" emphasizes the nontemporality of the intelligible act by which we freely choose the supreme maxim of our actions. The propensity to good or evil is "acquired" (if it is good) or "brought on us by ourselves" (if it is evil),[81] but it is not "acquired in time."[82] It is acquired or brought upon us because, as the authors of it, we are responsible for it; on the other hand, it is inborn because the responsibility for it arises from a choice made outside of time.

To emphasize this threefold characterization of the choice of a supreme maxim as radical, free, and nontemporal, Kant employs a somewhat odd expression: we are good or evil "by nature";[83] or again, the disposition by which the whole use of our freedom is determined is ours "by nature."[84] A phrase like this must surprise the reader accustomed to take the term "nature" as the exact opposite of what is designated by "freedom."[85] Whatever belongs to nature, or is dependent on nature, is subject to natural necessity. The entire problematic of the third antinomy consisted in showing how an action could be free even while being rigorously determined within a causal series. Thus the expression "by nature" may well generate confusion. Yet Kant is aware of this, and hastens to dispel any equivocalness by making plain that by the nature of man he means only "the subjective ground of the exercise (under objective moral laws) of man's freedom in general."[86] This ground must itself always be an act of freedom. Thus, in an astonishing reversal of Kant's terminology, the term "nature" receives a meaning altogether different from that

which ordinarily is attached to it and comes to designate freedom—
not any freedom, of course, but quite specifically the *finite* freedom
of a created rational being which has the power to determine itself
with respect to a freely chosen supreme maxim. Hence, it is correct
to consider the radical disposition of the human being "a property
of the will [*Willkür*] which belongs to it by nature [*von Natur
zukommt*],"[87] that is, ultimately, "a property of freedom which belongs to it by freedom."[88] If we can be called *morally* good or bad, it is
only because the "*natural* propensity"[89] to good or evil "must spring
from freedom"[90] and "must . . . be sought in a will [*Willkür*] which is
free."[91] "This propensity is so deeply rooted in the will [*Willkür*] that
we are forced to say that it is to be found in man by nature."[92]

We must not attribute this natural propensity to a nature which
is *given* but rather to the intelligible character of a nature which the
human being *gives itself* by an act of its freedom. By nature we are not
moral beings at all: we are neither morally good nor morally evil by
nature.[93] The character we adopt for ourselves can only be qualified
morally because it is the result of a free choice; we ourselves are the
authors of it. If we are good or bad, the credit or blame for it certainly must not be ascribed to nature.[94] When we speak of character,
"it does not depend on what Nature makes of man, but what man
makes of himself."[95]

From this perspective the essential distinction Kant establishes
between the propensity (*Hang*) and the predispositions (*Anlagen*) of
human nature stands out with particular clarity. While the propensity defines what we make of ourselves, the predispositions constitute "the possibility of human nature":[96] they determine the manner
in which nature makes us. These predispositions are three in num-
ber. The first concerns man as a living being endowed with a physical
self-love which he directs to preserve his life, to propagate the species, and to associate with others in forming a society. The second
treats the humanity of man as a living being who is also rational, and
as such endowed with a self-love which, illuminated by reason, he
directs to the acquisition of personal worth in the opinion of others.
The third considers man as a moral being and is nothing but his capacity for respect for the moral law, taken as an incentive in itself
adequate for free choice. Of these three original and indestructible
predispositions in human nature, which Kant calls "predispositions
toward good,"[97] insofar as they promote the realization of what is

good, clearly the third, in particular, deserves our attention.[98] This predisposition makes man a moral being *capable* of incorporating respect for the law into his maxims as a motive determining his action. In order to realize itself fully and to manifest its authentic autonomy, human freedom must not oppose nature but must surpass it: by actualizing in a free act a potentiality already inscribed in nature itself, by actually choosing the moral law as an incentive, that is, by *conjoining* the predisposition to good (*Anlage zum Guten*)[99] already constitutive of human nature to a propensity to good (*Hang zum Guten*), which would then indicate that the *Willkür* had decided to become *Wille*. "The original *predisposition* in man is good; not that, thereby, he is already actually good, but rather that he brings it about that he *becomes* [my emphasis] good or evil, according to whether he adopts or does not adopt into his maxim the incentives which this predisposition carries with it ([an act] which must be left wholly to his own free choice)."[100] Doubtless man is good by natural predisposition, but he will only be good "in actuality [*der That nach*]"[101] when he incorporates the moral law into his maxim as an incentive. It is certain that the structure for incorporating it is already in place, since a predisposition to the good which makes the determination of the will by the moral law possible can be found in human nature.[102] Hence the expression "predisposition to personality" which serves to designate this structure is particularly felicitous, since the notion of personality leads back directly to that of freedom, with which it is identified. "Moral personality is nothing but the freedom of a rational being under moral laws."[103]

The propensity is morally qualifiable, and in this way is distinguished from the natural predisposition, since it can be imputed to us.[104] It is "our own *act* [*That*]."[105] Yet is is not just any act; it is an "aboriginal act" preceding all sensible action. It is simply the nontemporal choice "whereby the supreme maxim (in harmony with the law or contrary to it) is adopted by the will [*Willkür*]."[106] Since this is a radical choice which determines the adoption of all secondary maxims, as well as all of our acts, it is not enough to say that it is *imputable* to us (*zurechnungsfähig*). We must also specify that this choice *grounds* all our judgments of imputability. Man is responsible for his actions—that much is beyond doubt. But whether his actions are those of a good or of a bad man is a question which evidently must remain unanswered, for, while the imputability is certain, the

judgments of imputability remain always contingent.[107] In order to
say that a man is evil, we would have to be in a position to observe
the ultimate disposition at the root of the bad acts done. But this is
impossible, for we can never be assured that a bad action really derives from a maxim which is itself bad. All maxims, even those
we choose ourselves, elude our observation. As a result, although we
know a priori that every man is responsible for the acts he does,
we can never know whether or not he is culpable when he does
something bad. Imputability is firmly grounded; our imputations are
not. "The judgement that the agent is an evil man cannot be made
with certainty if grounded on experience."[108] Note that Kant here
merely restates what he had already affirmed in the first *Critique* (see
pp. 38–39).

Our imputations apply only to empirical character. This is how
we are able to consider culpable those who, even from earliest child-
hood, evidence a precocious evil. We reproach them for their faults,
and such reproaches seem completely justified. But "this could not
happen if we did not suppose that whatever arises from man's choice
. . . has a free causality as its *ground,* which from early youth expresses its character in its appearances (its actions)."[109] Imputability is
thus grounded on the intelligible character. But the relation between
the two characters remains permanently unspecifiable, which explains why we are never permitted to draw conclusions about one
based on the other. The empirical character may even in certain
cases be good, while the intelligible character is radically evil, and
vice versa.[110] As Karl Jaspers says, "I can know only the legality of my
acts, never the morality of my intentions. I cannot know what I am
in truth; I cannot know if, having acted well, I have the right to consider myself good."[111]

If it were possible for us to know the intelligible character of a
man as it is revealed in sensible effects and, at the same time, all the
external circumstances which influence him, "his future conduct
could be predicted with as great a certainty as the occurrence of a
solar or lunar eclipse, [yet] we could . . . still assert that the man is
free."[112] The choice of intelligible character is a nontemporal choice
which determines the entirety of our actions in the phenomenal
order. Within the course of time, it seems that everything happens
as if there were no freedom. But can we conclude from the fact that
freedom is not internal to time that man is not free in the several

moments of his life? Kant's theory of freedom poses considerable difficulty on this point. We will attempt to overcome it by appeal to two levels of consideration.

In the first place, actions derived from the intelligible character certainly cannot be considered free actions themselves, since they are only appearances. In this regard, Schopenhauer was correct in affirming that Kant's theory of character is a translation of the famous scholastic formula, *Operari sequitur esse.* Freedom resides not in the *operari* but in the *esse.* In instituting the supreme maxim of his actions, man chooses his *esse,* and all his actions follow necessarily from this choice. Every man acts according to what he is. According to Schopenhauer, "Freedom appertains not to the empirical character, but only to the intelligible. The *operari* of a given person (what he does) is necessarily determined from without by the motives, and from within by his character; hence everything that he does necessarily takes place. In his *esse* (what he is), however, the freedom lies. He could have *been* a different man, and guilt or merit lies in what he is." [113] Responsibility rests with the *esse;* the *operari* fall under the sway of necessity. Every action is rigorously determined by the intelligible choice. The contingency of the act flows from the contingency of the choice. But once the choice is made, the act follows from it necessarily.

From this point of view, a rational being can rightly say of any unlawful action which he has done that he could have left it undone [*hätte unterlassen können*], even if as an appearance it was sufficiently determined in the past and thus far was inescapably necessary. For this action and everything in the past which determined it belong to a single phenomenon of his character, *which he himself creates* [*sich selbst verschafft*], and according to which he imputes to himself [*selbst zurechnet*] as a cause independent of all sensibility the causality of that appearance. [114]

Thus it is necessary to look to the *esse* to discover freedom. The question arises whether the being which I choose, which I give myself, is also free in each moment of its history. Must we consider the intelligible choice as a finished act? Must I think of my freedom as being wholly concentrated but also wholly exhausted in this act which is settled once and for all, so that my historical being is utterly fixed and determined by that choice? The being which is engaged in historical time is nevertheless, in part, disengaged from physical time: I am at once noumenon and phenomenon. The intelligible world is immanent within me. One must not claim to have been noumenal once and to be phenomenal now. The Platonic scheme laid down in the myth of Er the Pamphylian[115] must be strictly distinguished from Kant's theory and from the choice of an intelligible character. They can be compared only in order to see their contrast more clearly. The intelligible choice was not made in the past, prior to time, before the agent was subject to spatio-temporal determination. The choice is intelligible and nontemporal; yet the historical being is also intelligible and nontemporal, insofar as he is rational. We must claim, not that the choice of character *was made* before time, but that it *is made* outside of time and is nontemporal in this sense only. If the choice had been made before time, the *esse* would be fully determined by it and therefore would not be free at the present moment. It would have been free only at the moment of the choice by which it was constituted. In fact the past is no longer in my power; hence "every action which I perform is necessary because of determining grounds which are not in my power. That means that *at the time* [*Zeitpunkt*] I act I am never free."[116] Saying that the choice was made before time temporalizes it in a certain manner. But to the contrary, we must affirm that it is precisely because the choice is nontemporal that I can choose, in each moment, the being that I am. The moment must be conceived here as an "atom of eternity," or an "atom of non-temporality," disengaged from temporal determination, for otherwise it would be impossible to conceive it as the domain of freedom, since "every action which occurs at a certain point of time [*Zeitpunkt*] is necessary under the condition of what preceded it."[117] Because the choice is nontemporal, it is *unique*. I choose my being in every moment, not by a series of discrete choices, but by a single continuous choice. Doubtless the freedom of free choice is revealed by the freedom of indifference in a series of different choices. But this is not where intelligible freedom is empirically manifest. The moment assumes the aspect of nontemporality to the extent that, fully dependent of past and future, it forms an indivisible whole, a totality, like eternity itself. It is the privileged moment in time when the rational being reiterates its choice, when the freedom. In this way, Kant opposes the "use [*Gebrauch*]" of free choice (for good) to the "abuse [*Missbrauch*]" of free choice (for evil).[135] affirm, with Schopenhauer, that the agent is responsible for the acts he performs because "he could have *been* a different man."[118] On the contrary, we must say that the agent is responsible for his actions because he *can* be otherwise, for he chooses his being in each moment. The agent is free in every moment of his history to be what he is. On the other hand, since every agent acts according to what he is, we can assert that "it is *always* [*zu aller Zeit*] in everyone's power to satisfy the commands of the categorical command of morality."[119] The nontemporal choice does not consign me to determination by the past. The theory of character symbolizes our identity with ourselves both as unknown to ourselves and, nevertheless, as subtending each of our acts. Every phenomenal action can thus be conceived *sub specie aeternitatis:* when a man tells a lie, "the action is ascribed to the agent's intelligible character; in the *moment* when he utters the lie, the guilt is entirely his."[120] The liar was free and could have acted differently. "The act as well as its opposite must be within the power of the subject *at the moment* of its taking place [*in dem Augenblicke des Geschehens*]."[121] Thus, because it is the domain of freedom, the moment also appears as the time of regeneration. "However evil a man has been up to the very moment of an impending free act . . . it was not only his duty to have been better, it is *now* still his duty to better himself. To do so must be within his power, and if he does not do so, he is susceptible of, and subjected to, imputability [*Zurechnung*] *in the very moment* [my emphasis] of that action [*in dem Augenblicke der Handlung*], just as much as though . . . he had stepped out of a state of innocence into evil."[122] Freedom is always in acts.

The Choice of Radical Evil

The possibility of choosing a maxim which may either conform to or oppose the moral law evidences a weakness of freedom, insofar as it is incapable of determining itself solely in respect to the representation of the good. The actual choice by which I institute the supreme maxim of my actions is presented to me in the form of an alternative: I can be good *or* bad. If I choose the good, I fulfill both my freedom and the autonomy of my will. If I choose the bad, I suppress my freedom in some way and consign myself to heteronomy. In either case, however, the choice is a free act.

Man chooses evil. Indeed, the testimony of experience indicates that man is evil by nature. "That such a corrupt propensity must indeed be rooted in man need not be formally proved in view of the multitude of crying examples which experience *of the actions* of men

puts before our eyes."[123] However, the propensity to evil is not
analytically contained in the concept of man. Evil is contingent
[*zufällig*).[124] Yet we can still presuppose it as "*subjectively necessary* to
every man, even to the best."[125] As a result, the fact that man is "evil
by nature" means simply that "evil can be predicated of man as a
species."[126] This "*natural* propensity in man to evil"[127] cannot be
"represented as resulting from an already innate wickedness in our
nature."[128] It is contingent and "morally evil"[129] because it is a product of our free choice. "Hence a propensity to evil can inhere only in
the moral capacity of the will [*Willkür*]."[130] This choice is an *aboriginal*
fault (*peccatum originarium*),[131] which has its origin in reason and is
produced outside of time. It is not, properly speaking, an "*original*
sin,"[132] occurring at the beginning of time or at a particular moment
in the life of each man. "To seek the temporal origin of free acts as
such . . . is thus a contradiction. Hence it is also a contradiction to
seek the temporal origin [*Zeitursprung*] of man's moral character. . . .
In the search for the rational origin [*Vernunftursprung*] of evil actions,
every such action must be regarded as though [*als ob*] the individual
had fallen into it directly from a state of innocence. For whatever his
previous deportment may have been, . . . his action is yet free."[133]
The choice of evil is a personal choice, present at all times and in
every act, whereas the idea of a hereditary fault contradicts that of
freedom. "It is altogether legitimate," Kant says, "that man must
acknowledge the results of his actions as performed by himself, and
accept the full responsibility for all the evil that follows from the
abuse of his reason."[134] Thus, whoever chooses evil "abuses" his freedom. In this way, Kant opposes the "use [*Gebrauch*]" of free choice
(for good) to the "abuse [*Missbrauch*]" of free choice (for evil).[135]

Because free choice includes within itself an element of negativity
(insofar as it is not necessarily determined by the moral law), when it
in fact chooses a maxim which opposes the law it becomes a principle of negation. In the words of Nabert:

> Do we not often, in doctrines where free choice is most completely and
> categorically affirmed, admit a mystery—namely, the mystery of free-
> dom's deployment against itself? And do we not often specify the mystery
> further by recognizing a principle which limits the use of freedom inter-
> nally, or which at least explains how freedom can choose against its own
> best interest? It is sometimes said, doubtless correctly, that in introducing
> into human nature an incomprehensible propensity to evil arising from

free choice, Kant remains under the influence of specifically religious preoccupations. Yet we would rather consider this mystery evidence that doctrines of freedom can scarcely be maintained, since it tends (albeit through freedom) to reinstate a principle of negation.[136]

Such is the paradox of a freedom which disowns itself instead of fulfilling its essence. By choosing evil, freedom freely consigns itself to heteronomy. In a way, it annihilates itself. According to Kant, "We cannot see freedom in the act of a choice directed against the rational law."[137] Such, too, is the paradox of a reason which lays down the moral law, yet still chooses a maxim contrary to that law—which "originates" law,[138] yet is the source of the aboriginal fault.[139]

Moral evil thus remains incomprehensible to us for more than one reason. In the first place, evil is inexplicable because it arises from a free act, and "only events occurring according to the mechanism of nature are susceptible of explanation."[140] The choice of a supreme maxim is an "intelligible act [*intelligibele That*],"[141] which cannot be found in experience. Put another way, "Experience . . . never can reveal [*aufdecken*] the root of evil in the supreme maxim of the free will [*Willkür*] relating to the law, a maxim which, as *intelligible act*, precedes all experience."[142] Yet this is not just any intelligible act. It is an act we perform ourselves, but which nevertheless eludes our comprehension. "We can no more assign a further cause for the corruption in us by evil of just this highest maxim, although this is our own action, than we can assign a cause for any fundamental attribute belonging to our nature."[143] But is this true of every free act? If we confined ourselves to the reasons normally invoked to account for the inexplicable nature of moral evil, we would certainly understand why evil, just like the freedom from which it arises, is incomprehensible. But this course would leave an important aspect of the question obscure: evil results from freedom's absurd decision. Hence, it is yet more incomprehensible than freedom itself. The question of how reason can make an irrational choice, how freedom can render itself unfree, how the fundamental aim of the elective will can thwart that of the legislative will, how, ultimately, a propensity to evil (*Hang zum Bösen*) can be engendered in us when "the original predisposition . . . is a predisposition to good [*Anlage zum Guten*]"[144] constitutes the indecipherable paradox of ethics. "How actions contrary to the law occur remains inexplicable." [145] "Freedom can never be located in the fact that the rational subject is able to make a choice in opposition to his (legislative) reason, even though experience proves often enough that this does happen (though we cannot comprehend [*nicht begreifen können*] how this is possible)." [146] Since it is impossible for us to get beyond the subjective ground of the employment of our freedom, we cannot explain how evil is in us. The origin of evil remains "inscrutable" to us. [147] "Evil is *radical*, because it corrupts the ground of all maxims." [148] But this ground, this *Grund*, is itself without a ground (*Abgrund*), for "there is then for us no conceivable ground [*kein begreiflicher Grund*] from which the moral evil in us could originally have come." [149] We do not know what soil evil takes root in; it is conceived in an unfathomable deep.

The propensity to evil, which originates in man's free act, has three degrees: fragility, impurity, and wickedness. The fragility (*Gebrechlichkeit*) or weakness (*Schwäche*) of the heart is its inability in practice to follow the moral law which the will has incorporated into its maxim. The impurity (*Unlauterkeit*) of the heart consists in its tendency to appeal to extraneous incentives in order to determine its action in conformity with duty, rather than incorporating into its maxim the moral law as an adequate motive in itself. Finally, the wickedness (*Bösartigkeit*) or corruption (*Verderbtheit*) of the heart is precisely an inversion (*Verkehrtheit*), because it "reverses [*umkehrt*] the ethical order among the incentives of a *free* will [*Willkür*]." [150]

This threefold analysis exposes an enigma within Kant's philosophy as soon as we set it in the context of the rest of the *Religion,* where the propensity to evil is characterized as a reversal of the order of incentives in a maxim. Elsewhere it seems that only the third degree is important, so it is hard to see why Kant undertook to distinguish "three distinct degrees" within the propensity. [151] Then, too, is it not surprising that he describes the propensity to evil even before having established the reality of evil? Yet it is quite permissible to hold that for Kant this order of exposition, far from being arbitrary, [152] was justified and purposeful. If we succeed in deciphering this purpose, perhaps we will thereby also discover the solution to the enigma which this initially strange and ambiguous analysis poses.

It is important to recognize that this is not the first time we have seen Kant describe something given to consciousness before having established the effective reality of it. In this regard, a comparison with the *Grundlegung* seems particularly edifying. There Kant attempts to analyze the notion of duty as it appears in the judgment of popular consciousness before proving the objectivity of the concept. Similarly, in the *Religion* he examines human consciousness in order to describe how the propensity to evil he detects there subsists before asserting the existence of evil in every man. Consequently, the three degrees of that propensity amount to three descriptive levels of consciousness as it is lived. They suggest aspects of the propensity as it appears to consciousness without claiming to reveal what it is in itself or what its root is. At the first level, I acknowledge that by virtue of the autonomy of my will and of the primitive predisposition to the good which follows from it, the moral law exists in me as an incentive and urges me to do the good; nevertheless, I discover that "what I would, that I do not!"[153] At the second level, I note that when I perform a good action I do not necessarily act out of pure respect for the law. On the contrary, other sensuous motives are frequently (perhaps always) juxtaposed with the properly moral incentive. And these determine me to act in such manner that the collusion of egoistic motives with the moral incentive gives rise to good actions which in spite of being good have no moral character at all, since, although they conform to duty, they are not performed out of duty. Only the third descriptive level enables us to present the very essence of the propensity to evil as it will later be revealed in Kant's a priori analysis in the section devoted to the reality and origin of evil. The propensity to evil consists in a reversal of the moral order of the incentives we incorporate in our maxims. This means that ultimately the moral incentive is never merely juxtaposed with egoistic motives, but that it is subordinated to them. Depending on the circumstances, this subordination may result in actions which seem good when viewed externally, as well as in actions which are manifestly contrary to the law. Certainly my conscience clearly grasps the fundamental nature of this propensity to evil every time it experiences situations where there is no longer a collusion but rather a "clash"[154] between moral and sensuous motives, where the fortuitous juxtaposition of these motives no longer conceals the necessary subordination of the one to the other, where finally the deceptive complicity of the several motives yields to an overt conflict which can only end in the victory of one over the other. Thus, just as the good will is only revealed to the popular consciousness with full

clarity when it is struggling with the inclinations, the propensity to
evil as it is in itself is only present to consciousness when the inclinations engage in conflict with the moral law. On this point, too, the
comparison with the *Grundlegung* is evident. In order to identify the
good will, to be assured that the will acts out of duty and not by
inclination (*aus Neigung*), it is better to analyze those situations
where the will can only follow the moral law by renouncing the satisfaction of sensuous desires. Similarly, in order to identify the bad
will, to ascertain the priority it accords to sensuous motives over the
moral motive, it is better to examine those situations where the will
can only satisfy the inclinations by renouncing the moral law.

The origin of evil remains inscrutable. All we know is that the
principle of evil can be found neither in sensibility nor in the corruption of reason. It cannot be located in sensibility, for sensuous inclinations in themselves are neither good nor bad, and they are as
likely to further good as evil. Moreover, the inclinations are in us
without having been willed; how then could evil be imputable to us if
it had its ground in them? Man "does not even hold himself responsible for these inclinations and impulses or attribute them to his
proper self, i.e., his will, though he does ascribe to his will the indul-
gence which he may grant to them when he permits them an influence on his maxims to the detriment of the rational laws of his
will." [155] No more can evil be sought in a corruption (*Verderbnis*) of
legislative reason, since it would then be necessary to suppose that
reason had the power to destroy the moral legislation which by virtue of its own essence it must impose on itself. Such a supposition is
logically impossible. No free being can violate the law of freedom in a
pure spirit of revolt. "To conceive of oneself as a freely acting being
and yet as exempt from the law which is appropriate to such a thing
(the moral law) would be tantamount to conceiving a cause operating without any laws whatsoever (for determination according
to natural laws is excluded by the fact of freedom); this is a self-
contradiction." [156] Thus sensibility comprises too little to serve as the
principle of moral evil, since, if it could suppress the incentives
which arise from freedom, it would make man a purely *animal* being.
And reason comprises too much, since, if it could institute bare opposition to the moral law as an incentive, it would make man into a
demonic being. Yet man is neither beast nor devil.

This twofold orientation enables Kant to situate man's *evil* will in relation to the *brute* will and the *demonic* will. The nonrational animal is subject to strict natural determination; it is totally without freedom. Hence there can be no question of characterizing it morally. It is permissible to consider a particular animal evil by nature; yet it would be absurd to assert that it is "morally evil,"[157] for the idea of moral evil becomes self-contradictory when applied to an animal. Do we not then have good grounds to consider that what can be said about the animal applies *mutatis mutandis* to the demonic being? However strange it may seem, it would evidently be absurd to characterize a demonic being morally. That is, the idea of a demonic being, who chose evil for the sake of evil, appears as a limiting concept which destroys itself. To justify this assertion it is important to note that two distinct questions are concealed within this one problem, and these can be formulated in the following manner: (1) *Is* a demonic being endowed with freedom? (2) Can a being endowed with freedom *become* demonic?

In both cases the answer is no, so we can maintain that the demonic being is placed outside the domain of freedom, so to speak. That the demonic being cannot be free follows from the very notion of "malignant reason [*boshafte Vernunft*]," which is a self-contradictory notion, since it includes the idea of a reason set free from the very moral law which it must yet by virtue of its own essence lay down for itself. A malignant reason is one which, properly speaking, is disfigured; more, it is no longer quite reason. Indeed it is inconceivable that a reason could be free while divorced from the law of freedom. To answer the objection that for a rational causality to be bound necessarily to a law is clearly a mark of its finitude, and that it can only be presumed that a demonic being participates in this finitude, it is enough to recall that the moral law is universal. "This principle of morality . . . is declared by reason to be a *law for all rational beings* in so far as they have a will. . . . It is thus not limited to human beings but extends to all finite beings having reason and will; indeed, it includes the Infinite Being as the supreme intelligence."[158] Only finite reason is in a relation of *dependence* with respect to the moral law; nevertheless, all reason, whether finite or infinite, is *bound* to this law. A demonic being, therefore, could neither be rational nor free. Nor can we claim that the demonic being is one which is *no longer* rational, for such an assertion would leave open the possibility of a movement from a free state to a demonic state—a possibility

which Kant's analysis expressly excludes. On the one hand, a demonic being is not free; on the other hand, a free being cannot be
demonic. Thus evil constitutes a limit to freedom. One who is free
does not have the power to free himself from the law of freedom and
choose evil as such; freedom can never completely repudiate or an-
nihilate itself. A man can certainly disobey the moral law, but he
cannot make this disobedience into a determining motive for his will
(*Willkür*). "Man (even the most wicked) does not, under any maxim
whatsoever, repudiate the moral law in the manner of a rebel
[*rebellischerweise*] (renouncing obedience to it). The law, rather, forces
itself upon him irresistibly by virtue of his moral predisposition."[159]
The will is always legislative, and thus autonomous, even when the
particular choice of the will (*Willkür*) consigns us to heteronomy.[160]
There is no contradiction between the autonomy of the will and the
choice of radical evil, since "man acknowledges the authority of this
law even while transgressing it,"[161] and only transgresses it reluc-
tantly, "for there is no man so depraved but that he feels upon transgressing the internal law a resistance within himself and an abhor-
rence of himself."[162] Thus the human will is neither "absolutely . . .
good [*schlechterdings gut*],"[163] since it can choose evil, nor "absolutely
wicked [*schlechthin böser*],"[164] since it cannot choose evil as evil. It is
neither perfect, since it is not fully free, nor demonic, since it is free.

Radical evil is not absolute, yet it is something positive and not
derived from a mere lack. What then is this hostile motive which is
opposed to the positive principle of morality? As a being both rational and sensible, man incorporates into his maxim two incentives—that of the moral law and that of sensuous impressions. Since
his will cannot be irrational, the incentive of the moral law always
imposes itself on him and can never be excluded from his maxim.[165]
Evil, therefore, does not consist in the context of incentives but in
the manner in which they are subordinated to one another. Man becomes wicked when he inverts and corrupts the moral order of incentives, that is, when he subordinates the rational law to self-love as
a determining principle of the will.[166] He then obeys the moral law
only to the extent that it is useful to him in satisfying his sensuous
inclinations.[167] "He makes the incentive of self-love and its inclinations the condition of obedience to the moral law; whereas, on the
contrary, the latter, as the *supreme condition* of the satisfaction of the
former, ought to have been adopted into the universal maxim of

the will [*Willkür*] as the sole incentive."[168] Obedience to the unconditioned law is reduced "to the merely conditional character of a means."[169] What is really an end in itself becomes merely a means. The corruption of the human heart is the result of a free act which arises from reason, even though it is contrary to the legislative reason. Indeed it is reason itself which subordinates itself to the sensuous. The impairment by sensibility is produced in the realm of the intelligible. But reason as such is not corrupted, and remains legislative, since the moral law is still imposed on us. Hence we can conclude with Nabert that "relative to the duality of reason and sensibility, free will [*Willkür*], in Kant's thought, leaves the higher truth of a freedom adequate to reason intact."[170]

6   *Negation of the Negation: Regeneration*

Conversion

"Perversity of the heart," Kant claims, "may coexist with a will which in general is good."[1] Evil, that is, is not absolute evil. The human being is not "*basically* corrupt,"[2] since his will remains autonomous and legislative. Only with regret does he transgress the moral law. "In order to imagine the vicious person as tormented with mortification by the consciousness of his transgressions, [one] must presuppose that he is, in the core of his character, at least *to a certain degree morally good.*"[3] However, it must not be concluded that man is at once good and bad; insofar as the moral law is not re-established in its absolute purity, insofar as it is not accepted as the only adequate incentive and the sole determining principle of the will, man must be considered a wicked being. Nevertheless, he always preserves a feeling of respect for the law and, precisely because this "seed of goodness [*Keim des Guten*]"[4] abides in him in all its purity, a conversion is possible.

The possibility of such a conversion cannot be disputed; even in spite of our fall, the obligation to become better is imposed on us with equal force. Thus we must have the ability to submit to this obligation; it is forbidden to "content ourselves with repentence."[5] The possibility of conversion is deduced analytically from the positive concept of freedom. Kant affirms that evil must be able to be *overcome,* "since it is found in man, a being whose actions are free,"[6] yet evidently it is "*inextirpable* by human powers,"[7] since the ultimate subjective ground of all maxims is presumed to be corrupt. Perhaps we should conclude that the effectiveness of the propensity to evil, considered as *peccatum in potentia,*[8] is, so to speak, suspended, or paralyzed by our conversion in such a way that there would never be a movement from the capacity to the act. In fact, a quite radical regeneration is required in order to deliver us from radical evil. Conversion consists essentially in a reinstitution of "the original moral order among the incentives."[9] "The conversion of the disposition of a bad man into that of a good one is to be found in the change of the highest inward ground of the adoption of all his maxims, conformable to the moral law, so far as this new ground . . . is now itself unchangeable."[10] This conversion, therefore, will not result in progressive reform, but instead in a genuine moral revolution. Hence, we must undoubtedly acknowledge that the propensity to evil can really be extirpated, even though we should necessarily conceive of it as "ineradicable [*unvertilgbar*]."[11] The intellect is required to admit the possibility of regeneration without being able to explain it.

The moral law is nothing but the decree which the objective will directs to the subjective will in commanding its own reinstatement. The conversion to the good, which is imposed on us by our legislative will (*Wille*), is attributable to our free choice (*Willkür*). "Man *himself* must make or have made himself into whatever, in a moral sense, whether good or evil, he is or is to become. Either condition must be an effect of his free choice [*Willkür*]; for otherwise he could not be held responsible for it and could therefore be *morally* neither good nor evil."[12] Both the choice of evil and the conversion to the good are the work of our free choice. They arise from the same nontemporal choice by which we determine the law of the causality of our will. The immutability of intelligible character, as we have seen, pertains to time and in no way excludes the possibility of a modification in the free determination of freedom (see pp. 33–35). Therefore an alteration of our character is possible; this alteration must be conceived as independent of every relation to time, however, since it arises from an intelligible act. As Nabert observes:

> One celebrates victory prematurely in charging Kant with a contradiction between the idea of a conversion which includes the difference between before and after and the affirmation of the nontemporal character of conversion. For the demarcation of before and after symbolizes and expresses temporally the act of choosing between contrary maxims—maxims whose creation is itself an act of freedom. Yet since the free, rational act which effects our regeneration is not a step by step reformation, we call it nontemporal.[13]

Moreover, even though this intelligible act may be symbolized in sensuous life by a continual progress towards the good, it is unknowable. Just as the empirical character cannot give us knowledge of the intelligible character, moral progress, which we will eventually be able to discern in our sensuous life, cannot assure us of the authenticity of our regeneration. Thus, while our original corruption is absolutely certain, our conversion remains always problematic.

One result of the preceding analysis is that, in characterizing the autonomy of that will which obeys the moral law, we should affirm that this autonomy, too, remains problematic. Still, in calling the will (*Wille*) which institutes moral legislation autonomous, we affirm that the human will, as a pure will, *is* always autonomous, since it cannot be diabolical. These are the two aspects of the autonomy of the human will (see pp. 78–79). Under the first aspect, autonomy is problematic because the *accomplishment* of our moral revolution is always uncertain. Under the second aspect, autonomy (which cannot be challenged) grounds the *possibility* of our regeneration. "For man, therefore, who despite a corrupted heart yet possesses a *good will,* there remains *hope* of a return to the good from which he has strayed."[14]

This "hope" (*Hoffnung*) is well grounded, since the possibility of our regeneration is certain. But it will never be transformed into knowledge, nor even into belief, for the realization of our moral renewal always remains problematic. The human being can never know with certainty if he has really reestablished the moral arrangement of incentives in his maxim. In his own eyes his conversion always remains doubtful. "Yet he must be able to *hope* [*muss er hoffen können*] through his *own* efforts [*durch eigene Kraftanwendung*] to reach the road which leads thither."[15]

If our regeneration were not the work of our freedom, good could not be imputed to us. Kant remarks that Spener deserved credit for maintaining that the human being must not merely become better but that he must become different. But he was wrong to believe that this radical renovation was possible only with divine assistance. "Since the *supersensible* [*Übersinnliche*] in us is inconceivable and yet practical, we can well excuse those who are led to consider it *supernatural* [*übernatürlich*]—that is, to regard it as the influence of another and higher spirit, something not within our power and not belonging to us as our own. Yet they are greatly mistaken in this."[16] Spener made the mistake of believing that a miracle was necessary to realize that which in fact must result from the power of our practical reason. Strictly speaking, Kant's thought here tends toward Pelagianism.

Nevertheless, he is too conscious of the limits of human reason to adhere to Pelagius's doctrine without reservation. It may be, he grants, that divine assistance is required to compensate for the inadequacy of our power and to permit us to attain to the good. "For man must be able to become what his vocation requires him to be (adequate to the holy law); and if he cannot do this naturally by his own power, he may hope to achieve it by God's cooperation from without (whatever form this may take)." [17] What is certain is that each human being must, with respect to his efforts, do his best to become better; each must bring his talents to fruition. Only under these conditions "can he *hope* that what is not within his power will be supplied through cooperation from above." [18] In striving to follow the moral law, we "render ourselves susceptible of higher, and for us inscrutable, assistance." [19] What matters for us as human beings is not knowing exactly what this help consists in, but knowing what we ought to do "to become worthy of this assistance." [20] Hence, Kant admits the possibility of divine assistance; nevertheless, this assistance remains problematic in two ways. In the first place, we do not know if divine grace is truly necessary. Although we are aware of our limits, we have no proof of the insufficiency of our abilities for the duty laid on us; we can still hope to become good by our own efforts. In the second place, supposing that our power was indeed insufficient, we have no proof that it would be made good by divine grace; we can only hope to receive God's assistance. We are not, however, unaware that the conditions of the possibility of this supernatural aid must be fulfilled by the power of our freedom, which must make us "worthy of this assistance" [21] and "allow divine grace to act in us" [22] if we should receive it. In short, divine assistance is problematic both because we can "hope" to accomplish our moral renewal "through [our] *own* efforts" [23] and because we can only "hope that what is not within [our] power will be supplied through cooperation from above." [24] On the other hand, there can be no doubt that in every case the conversion to the good springs from our free choice and must be imputable to us.

Granted that some supernatural cooperation may [also] be necessary to his becoming good, or to his becoming better, yet, whether this cooperation consists merely in the abatement of hindrances or indeed in positive assistance, man must first make himself worthy to receive it, and must *lay hold* [*annehmen*] of this aid (which is no small matter)—that is, he must adopt this positive increase of power into his maxim [*in seine Maxime aufnehmen*], for only thus can good be imputed to him and he be known as a good man.[25]

The Postulate of Freedom

"Can God give man a good will? No, for a good will requires freedom." [26] It is up to us, and us alone, whether we shall be moral beings or not. God can certainly create us insofar as we are natural beings, but He cannot make virtuous beings of us. To attain to the good we can rely only on our own efforts and not on divine grace. It is man's dignity that he owes his perfection only to himself. What does this perfection consist in if not precisely in obedience to the moral law which the categorical imperative (an imperative which doubtless would lose all sense if we could not conform to it) imposes on him? The demand of duty always implies the consciousness of an ability. Thus, despite the universality of evil—which extends throughout the entire race—and by virtue of the obligation imposed on every human being to "become better," [27] it is necessary to presuppose "the capacity (*facultas*) to overcome all opposing sensible impulses . . . on behalf of freedom." [28]

At this stage of our analysis it is appropriate to bring in the postulate of freedom as Kant presents it in the Dialectic of the second *Critique*. This postulate, he asserts, "comes from the necessary presupposition [*notwendigen Voraussetzung*] of independence from the world of sense and of the capacity [*des Vermögens*] of determining man's will by the law of an intelligible world." [29] Everything occurs as if in the Critical Elucidation of the Analytic of Pure Practical Reason (a section placed between the Analytic and the Dialectic) Kant had foreseen the problem of evil and had been led thereby to introduce a new concept of freedom into his system at the level of the Dialectic. For this reason it seemed legitimate to make a detour through the doctrine of radical evil before approaching the question of the postulate of freedom. We shall see that the meaning of this postulate fully justifies the path we have followed.[30] In addition, we should not be led into error by the chronology of Kant's works. Certainly the "Essay on Radical Evil" in the *Religion* appeared only in 1793, but "the insurmountable wickedness of our heart" [31] had already long haunted him, as the 28 April 1775 letter to Lavater testifies.[32]

It remains no less true that the postulate of freedom originates in the body of the critical elucidation of the dialectic which affects pure practical reason, not in a reflection on radical evil. "In both its speculative and its practical employment, pure reason always has its dialectic, for it demands the absolute totality of conditions for a given conditioned thing, and this can be reached only in things-in-themselves."[33] Yet while the demand of the unconditioned in the speculative domain engenders an illusion (*Schein*) as inevitable as it is natural (in particular, the illusion of freedom), the same rational demand authorizes us to postulate its own realization in the practical domain, together with the conditions of the possibility of its realization (among which freedom figures prominently). Thus one of the two dialectics succeeds precisely where the other fails. How can we account for a similar difference in the manner of treating these two conflicts of reason?

The unconditioned totality which pure practical reason demands consists in the highest good, that is, "the whole, the perfect good [*ganz und vollendete*],"[34] which is only realized when morality is added to happiness. Thus, according to the formula of Paul Ricoeur, "practical reason . . . requires to be added to the object of its aim, that this object may be whole, what it excluded from its principles, that they might be pure."[35] But this aim (*die Absicht auf das höchste Gut*)[36] is itself imposed on our will by the moral law (*der alleinige Bestimmungsgrund des reinen Willens*).[37] "The moral law alone must be seen as the ground for making the highest good and its realization or promotion the object of the pure will."[38] "The moral law commands us to make the highest possible good in a world the final object of all our conduct."[39] This explains the fruitfulness of the dialectic of practical reason, which opens up perspectives on the intelligible world which were forbidden in the theoretical domain. Whereas on the plane of knowledge pure speculative reason correctly demanded the unconditioned without legitimately being able to claim to satisfy that demand (because of the finitude of the mind lacking strictly intellectual intuition), in the domain of action, pure practical reason must be able to satisfy its demand for the unconditioned, since that demand is guaranteed by a "fact [*Factum*]" which is nothing but the moral law itself. The realization of the highest good "is an a priori necessary object of our will and is inseparably related to the moral law."[40] To maintain that this realization is impossible would amount to considering the moral law "as the mere deception of our reason,"[41] and this cannot be. The moral law cannot be "fantastic, directed to empty imaginary ends, and consequently inherently false,"[42] since it is a fact of pure reason to which apodictic certainty adheres. As a result, the highest good must be possible.[43]

Consequently, it is not a question of knowing *if* the highest good is practically possible, but *how* it is possible.[44] It is the task of a critical philosophy to distinguish the conditions of the possibility of the object of the will—to make clear what common reason grasps only more or less obscurely. "I must presuppose [the object's] possibility and also its conditions, which are God, freedom, and immortality."[45] The belief in the infinite duration of my being grants me the assurance that, thanks to the power of my freedom, I can make indefinite progress towards a perfect morality; but only the belief in the existence of God guarantees me that happiness will be brought into a perfect proportion with morality to constitute the highest good.[46] Here, then, the three supreme objects of metaphysics—freedom, immorality, and God (whose objective reality cannot be assured by pure speculative reason)—are postulated through the moral law and receive a degree of reality through an exclusively practical employment. In this way the metaphysics according to ethics, which Kant had outlined in the Analytic of Practical Reason when he proved the objective reality of freedom, is elaborated at the level of the Dialectic (see pp. 67–70). Is it not also astonishing that we rediscover the freedom which was proven starting from the moral law at the level of the postulates? Is it in fact the same freedom? Before attempting to answer this question, it will first be helpful to analyze the very notion of a postulate.

A postulate of pure practical reason is "a *theoretical* proposition which is not as such demonstrable, but which is an inseparable corollary [*unzertrennlich anhängt*] of an a priori unconditionally valid *practical* law."[47] Postulates are theoretical propositions, for they pertain to things which exist; nevertheless, they are not "theoretical dogmas,"[48] which claim to extend our speculative knowledge, but rather "theoretical hypotheses,"[49] which must be admitted for the sake of the practical employment of our reason. As we have seen, "it is a duty to realize the highest good as far as it lies within our power to do so; therefore, it must be possible to do so. Consequently, it is unavoidable for every rational being in the world to assume whatever is necessary to its objective possibility. The assumption

[*Voraussetzung*] is as necessary [*notwendig*] as the moral law, in relation to which alone it is valid." [50] Therefore a postulate is a "necessary assumption [*notwendige Annehmung*]," [51] or a "necessary theoretical hypothesis." [52] But what sort of necessity is involved? It would seem that we can characterize it in three different ways. It is a matter of *logical necessity*. "In order not to come into contradiction with itself," [53] and "to think in a way consonant with morality," [54] practical reason, which orders us to seek to realize the highest good, must grant the conditions which alone make that realization possible. "Reason cannot command one to follow a purpose which is cognized as nothing more than a chimera." [55] Yet precisely this demand for logical coherence rests on a law decreed by practical reason. In other words, logical necessity has recourse to a "moral necessity" [56] as its ground; it is morally necessary to admit the existence of God, immortality, and freedom. It is "a necessity connected with duty as a requisite." [57] Reason is not only anxious to preserve its own coherence, [58] it is also (and more immediately) animated by the need to keep its promises. "For a final purpose cannot be commanded by any law of reason without this latter at the same time promising, however uncertainly, its attainableness, and thus justifying our belief [*Fürwahrhalten*] in the special conditions under which alone our reason can think it as attainable." [59] By giving our free assent to these postulates, we express our "trust in the promise of the moral law"; [60] and our belief in this promise is properly called a "rational faith [*Vernunftglaube*]," [61] because, in effect, it concerns a faith rooted in pure reason and derived from the moral purpose. [62] "Faith (absolutely so called) is trust in the attainment of a design, the promotion of which is a duty, but the possibility of the fulfillment of which (and consequently also that of the only conditions of it thinkable by us) is not to be *comprehended* by us." [63] This explains how the need of pure practical reason, unlike that of pure reason in its speculative employment, leads us not only to hypotheses but also to postulates. The former need is "based on a duty" [64] (that of working towards the realization of the highest good) and is, as a result, "unconditional." [65] We must not say that we are compelled to suppose the existence of God, immortality, and freedom *if* we want to realize the highest good but *because we ought* to strive to realize it. [66] "This is, therefore, an absolutely necessary need [*ein Bedürfnis in schlechterdings notwendiger Absicht*] and justifies its presupposition not merely as an allowable hypothesis but as a practical postulate."[67] The necessity of admitting the conditions of the highest good is grounded on a duty,[68] but "this moral necessity is subjective, i.e., a need, and not objective, i.e., duty itself,"[69] for there cannot be a duty to admit the existence of a thing. "Faith that is commanded is an absurdity [*Unding*]."[70] Hence this moral necessity is a "subjective" necessity,[71] a necessity known "with reference to the subject,"[72] which bears no "theoretical," "apodictic,"[73] or "*logical*" certainty,[74] but merely a "*moral* certainty."[75] "I must not even say, '*It is* morally certain that there is a God, etc.,' but '*I am* morally certain, etc.'"[76] Rational faith implies a movement at once personal and free.[77]

From here it is possible to indicate the status of the freedom postulated in Kant's philosophy. Certainly he never specified the relation which binds this notion of freedom together with that which was deduced analytically from the moral law, and his thinking on this point displays an equivocation which it is important to clear up. How can we explain the fact that Kant, having once granted freedom a privileged place among the ideas of pure speculative reason (see pp. 67–70), now locates it at the level of the postulates, that is, at the same level as the ideas of God and immortality?[78] Our analysis of the notion of the postulate allows us to presume that we are here in the presence of two forms of freedom which must be carefully distinguished. It is appropriate to note at the outset that the freedom which is proved (*beweisen*) by the law,[79] in the Analytic, and that which is merely postulated (*postuliert*) by the law,[80] in the Dialectic, are installed in the structure of Kant's work quite differently. While the former is "the condition of the moral law,"[81] the latter is one of the conditions of the possibility of the highest good,[82] that is, one of the conditions which make the accomplishment of the necessary object prescribed by the moral law possible. Just as the moral law grounds the idea of the highest good, the autonomy of the will is the ground of the postulates of practical reason. These two notions of freedom, therefore, are not on the same level. The first is a *fact* of practical reason; the second is a *postulate* of practical reason. The one is the legislative power of a will which institutes the moral law; the other is the practical power of a will capable of following that law. It is freedom understood as autonomy of the will which enjoys a place of privilege among the ideas of pure reason. On one side, it allows us to grant objective reality to the ideas of God and immortality; on the other side, it must be ranked, not among the *Glaubenssachen* (*res fidei*), but among the *Thatsachen* (*res facti*)—not among the *credibilia,* but among the *scibilia.* The freedom which is postulated, on the other hand, is a "pure *rational faith* [*Vernunftglaube*]"[83] and as such can be numbered among the *Glaubenssachen.*[84] We know (*wissen*) that reason commands our obedience to duty; we believe (*glauben*) that we have the ability to act out of duty. Since the freedom which is postulated is, like all the other postulates, grounded on the moral law (that is, ultimately, on freedom as the *ratio essendi* of the law), we cannot attribute to it the same *indubitable* objective reality (see pp. 59–61)[85] which we ought to acknowledge in the freedom which is proved by the law. The only certainty which belongs to it is a "moral certainty."[86]

Without doubt it was useful to appeal to Kant's terminology, and to consider the very structure of the second *Critique* before attempting to extract the underlying meaning of the postulate of freedom. Here we can refer to Delbos's excellent interpretation. "Freedom, as Kant considers it here, in the Dialectic of Practical Reason (where it is not identical to the law but 'postulated through the law'), is not the capacity of the pure will for being autonomous or for instituting universal legislation but the power vested in the subject for accomplishing its moral task under the authority of that legislation."[87] The passages which confirm this interpretation are so numerous as to seem decisive. The freedom which is postulated through the law is nothing but "a capacity [*Vermögen*] for following the moral law with an unyielding disposition."[88] It is this faculty which Kant will later name the autocracy of freedom. Discussing the three ideas of pure reason in the *Progress,* Kant remarks that, in addition to the autonomy of the legislative will, the idea of freedom includes autocracy. "That is, even here in earthly life, amidst all the hindrances that the influences of nature may place upon us as sensible creatures, still at the same time as intelligible beings this autocracy is assumed as the ability to achieve what pertains to the formal condition of freedom, morality."[89] In the *Verkündigung des nahen Abschlusses eines Tractats zum ewigen Frieden in der Philosophie,* freedom, considered as a postulate under the same rubric as God and immortality, is defined as the "capacity in a man of insuring the fulfillment of his duties (as if those duties were divine commandments) in the face of every natural power."[90] Finally, in the *Metaphysical Principles of Virtue,* Kant specifies that the distinction between autonomy and autocracy is justified by the finitude of human freedom.

For finite holy beings (who cannot even be tempted to violate duty) there is no doctrine of virtue, but only a doctrine of morals; this is so because the doctrine of morals is an autonomy of practical reason, while the doctrine of virtue is at the same time an autocracy of practical reason. This is to say, such autocracy contains a consciousness—although not immediately perceived, yet nevertheless rightly inferred from the moral categorical imperative—of the power to become master of one's inclinations that oppose the law.[91]

What can we distill from our encounter with these texts? Freedom as a postulate, or autocracy, is the capacity the human being possesses of fulfilling the moral task in *this* world. It is essentially the freedom of historical being. It is not so much "free choice regenerated,"[92] as Delbos calls it, as it is the capacity for regenerating free choice. While it may be, like all freedom, an extramundane causality, it is exercised "even here in earthly life."[93] It is in each instant of our lives that we, as rational beings, have the possibility of modifying the choice of our intelligible character. This freedom is directly connected to intelligible free choice, yet it is distinguished from it to the extent that it only overcomes being because our free choice is *initially* wicked. Since the wicked free choice in a sense denies its freedom, by subordinating reason to sensibility, and since only that free choice which is determined by virtue of rational principles is genuinely free, we can say that autocracy is our free capacity for reclaiming the freedom of our free choice, for entering once again into possession of our true *"free* will [*freien Willkür*]."[94] This is the power, which every human being possesses, of combating the propensities of his nature and "*conquering* them by means of reason, not in the future, but *right now* [*gleich jetzt*] (simultaneously with the thought)."[95] Thus it is a will stamped with the character of struggle, a "militant freedom,"[96] which is directly opposed to the corruption of our will. It must be possible for us, if not to "extirpate [*vertilgen*]," at least to "dominate [*überwiegen*]"[97] the propensity to evil, and to make ourselves "master of [those] inclinations that oppose the law."[98] Virtue is "moral disposition *in conflict*."[99] Grounded on the autonomy of our legislative will, autocracy is nothing but our capacity for realizing this autonomy by submitting to the rational law. It is to this form of freedom that the formula, "You ought, therefore you can," applies most precisely. We believe we have the capacity to act out of duty, and that belief is a need of the reason which has the force of law, since casting doubt on that capacity would cast doubt on the moral law itself.[100] Thus, while our conversion (which always remains problematic) is an object of *hope,* the capacity to convert ourselves is an object of rational *faith.*

Conclusion to Part II

Despite the diversity of forms described in it, Kant's doctrine of freedom presents a quite remarkable unity. Without doubt it presents certain obscurities and imprecisions, yet the difficulties it raises can be surmounted, provided we consider the Kantian domain in its entirety rather than one or another particular work. Thus, throughout this analysis it has seemed to us that the different concepts of freedom are rigorously bound to one another and form a coherent and harmonious whole. By laying out their genealogy, we have been able to observe how all these concepts converge on the notion of the autonomy of the will, the true keystone of the critical system.

But what good is it to extract the expressions of different concepts within a system? It may well be granted that an attempt to illuminate the logical coherence of the system is a useful enterprise, and it will certainly be acknowledged that this is an indispensable preliminary task, at least if we seek to penetrate the heart of the thought. But is this the only benefit we can hope to acquire from the present study? Must we resign ourselves to admitting that our entire reflection is limited to setting out the logical structure of the doctrine while cautiously avoiding any pronouncement about its value? Perhaps it is not appropriate for us to judge it ourselves. Nevertheless, we can say that in undertaking the work our aim was not to dissect a system, as anatomists dissect a cadaver, but to bring out the natural expressions of a body of thought which remains both vital and contemporary. For the problem of the coherence of Kant's doctrine of freedom leads us back to another question which, for us, is yet more decisive and fundamental: Why did Kant present freedom under such different aspects? By undertaking to answer this question, we believe we have shown that the complexity of Kant's analysis is simply a faithful reflection of the complexity which inheres in the very essence of human freedom.

The notion of autonomy of the will adequately expresses the freedom of the infinite being; the divine will is fully free precisely because it is necessarily determined to follow the moral law. It is not the same with the human being—a being which is rational but finite. When we consider the essence of his being as free, we witness the idea of freedom breaking through in a wide diversity of notions. Reason must be sought, on one side, in the finitude of our being and, on the other side, in its unhappy destiny.

The human will, which is autonomous insofar as it has a purely rational essence, is also affected by sensuous motives. Man's dual citizenship in the intelligible and the sensible worlds obliges us to distinguish in him a legislative autonomous will (*Wille*), an intelligible freedom of choice (*Willkür*) relative to both reason and sensibility, and a freedom of indifference—the empirical manifestation of this free choice. The human will as *Wille* wills the law. But as *Willkür* it can also not will the law. This noncoincidence of the self with itself testifies to the finitude of the being for whom obedience to the moral law does not necessarily accompany the laying down of that law by autonomous reason. The human being is destined, but not determined, to the good; the ability to deviate from the moral law, which is certainly not a necessary characteristic of freedom, is in reality only an incapacity. Man's whole moral task consists in acting in such a way that his *Willkür* becomes *Wille,* so that the initial disharmony which characterizes him in his finitude may be overcome. It is the duty of the human being to become autonomous.

The history of freedom begins with evil. By choosing to subordinate the moral law to sensuous motives, the human being, far from overcoming the division in his own will, only confirms it and henceforth assumes all responsibility for it; for if the finitude of his being cannot be imputed to him, he nevertheless freely chooses his being and his destiny. In other words, the incapacity of our free choice (the possibility of transgressing the moral law) is a negation which results from the unavoidable finitude of our being, while the choice of radical evil (the act of transgressing the moral law) is a privation resulting from a contingent act of our freedom.

Nevertheless, the history of human freedom, which is set down by freedom itself, is not merely the history of its deposition; it is also the history of its possible reinstatement. For there is in fact no genuine symmetry between good and evil; even when he chooses evil, the finite rational being remains destined to the good. It is always his duty to become autonomous, but he cannot become demonic: he has the ability to act out of pure respect for the law, and to choose the good for the sake of the good, but not to choose evil for the sake of evil. Whereas there is a limit to freedom in evil, there is none in the good. The doctrine of the postulates tells us that freedom can surpass every assigned limit, and the progress towards holiness can be continued indefinitely. The chief characteristic of the rational faith in freedom is never to separate the fall into evil from a possible conversion to the good.

Abbreviations

Passages from Kant's most frequently cited texts are from the following editions, and are referred to by the following abbreviations. Other citations from Kant's works have been taken from the standard edition of his *Werke: Kant's gesammelte Schriften* (hrsg. Königlich Preussischen Akademie der Wissenschaften [Berlin: Georg Reimer Verlag]), cited in notes as Ak. with volume and page numbers.

Anthropology   *Anthropology From a Pragmatic Point of View.* Translated by Victor Lyle Dowdell. Carbondale, Ill.: Southern Illinois University Press, 1978.

C.F.J.   *Kant's Critique of Judgment.* Translated by J. H. Bernard. New York: Hafner Publishing Company, 1951.

C.P.R.   *Immanuel Kant's Critique of Pure Reason.* Translated by Norman Kemp Smith. London: Macmillan Press, 1929.

C.Pr.R.   *Critique of Practical Reason.* Translated by Lewis White Beck. Indianapolis: Bobbs-Merrill Company, 1956.

Confl. Fac.   *The Conflict of the Faculties.* Translated by Mary J. Gregor. New York: Abaris Books, 1979.

Diss.   *Kant's Inaugural Dissertation of 1770.* Translated by John Handyside. Chicago: Open Court Publishing Company, 1928.

Education   *Education.* Translated by Annette Churton. Ann Arbor: University of Michigan Press, 1960.

F.M.M.   *Foundations of the Metaphysics of Morals.* Translated by Lewis White Beck. Indianapolis: Bobbs-Merrill Company, 1959.

Logic   *Logic.* Translated by Robert S. Hartman and Wolfgang Schwarz. Indianapolis: Bobbs-Merrill Company, 1974.

M.P.R.   *The Metaphysical Principles of Right.* In *The Metaphysical Principles of Virtue.* Indianapolis: Bobbs-Merrill Company, 1964.

M.P.V.   *The Metaphysical Principles of Virtue.* Translated by James Ellington. Indianapolis: Bobbs-Merrill Company, 1964.

Progress   *What Real Progress Has Metaphysics Made in Germany since the*

Time of Leibniz and Wolff? Translated by Ted Humphrey. New York: Abaris Books, 1983.

Proleg.   *Prolegomena to any Future Metaphysics.* Translated by Paul Carus. Revised by Paul Ellington. Indianapolis: Hackett Publishing Company, 1977.

Religion   *Religion within the Limits of Reason Alone.* Translated by Theodore M. Greene and Hoyt H. Hudson. New York: Harper & Row, 1960.

Theory-Practice *On the Old Saw: That May Be Right in Theory but It Won't Work in Practice.* Translated by E. B. Ashton. Philadelphia: University of Pennsylvania Press, 1974.

Notes

Introduction

1. *C.Pr.R.*, p. 107; Ak. 5:103.
2. Ibid., p. 109; Ak. 5:105.
3. Ibid., p. 8; Ak. 5:7.
4. *C.P.R.*, p. 424; Ak. A466=B494.
5. *C.Pr.R.*, p. 3; Ak. 5:3.
6. V. Delbos, *La philosophie pratique de Kant*, 3rd ed. (Paris: Presses Universitaires de France, 1969), p. 158.
7. Ibid. We have thought it appropriate to limit our subject to an examination of these problems without developing the conception of freedom as it appears in Kant's political thought. For a study of his political thought, see G. Vlachos, *La pensée politique de Kant* (Paris: Presses Universitaires de France, 1962) and A. Philonenko, *Théorie et praxis dans la pensée morale et politique de Kant et de Fichte en 1793* (Paris: Vrin, 1968).
8. "If we take single passages, torn from their contexts, and compare them with one another, apparent contradictions are not likely to be lacking, especially in a work that is written with any freedom of expression. In the eyes of those who rely on the judgment of others, such contradictions have the effect of placing the work in an unfavourable light; but they are easily resolved by those who have mastered the idea of the whole" (*C.P.R.*, p. 37; Ak. Bxliv). This remark is in general true of every oeuvre and not merely of particular texts or works.

Chapter One

1. *Progress*, p. 109; Ak. 20:287.
2. *C.P.R.*, pp. 409–14; Ak. A445–51=B473–79.
3. Ibid., p. 257; Ak. A235=B294.
4. Ibid.
5. Ibid., p. 411; Ak. A447=B475.
6. Ibid., p. 218; Ak. B232. In the second analogy of experience Kant showed that an event cannot be isolated, nor can it ever be understood without reference to other events. An event names a series. "That something happens, i.e., that something, or some state which did not previously exist, comes to be, cannot be perceived unless it is preceded by an appear-

ance which does not contain in itself this state. For an event which should follow upon an empty time, that is, a coming to be preceded by no state of things, is as little capable of being apprehended as empty time itself. Every apprehension of an event is therefore a perception that follows upon another perception" (*C.P.R.*, pp. 220–21; Ak. A191–92=B236–37). Precisely because an event is set in a causal series, in a linkage of cause and effect, it is necessarily objective; indeed, if it were not so, "we should then have only a play of representations, relating to no object" (*C.P.R.*, p. 222; Ak. A194=B239).

7. *Proleg.*, p. 84; Ak. 4:343–44 (my emphasis).

8. *C.P.R.*, p. 410; Ak. A444=B472.

9. Ibid., p. 411; Ak. A446=B472. If an event names a series (see n. 6 above), the series itself must be completed. The completion of the series answers to a demand of reason for "the *unconditioned*, which reason, of necessity and by right, *demands* [my emphasis] in things in themselves, as required to *complete* [my emphasis] the series of conditions" (*C.P.R.*, p. 24; Ak. Bxx). The entire problem of the Transcendental Dialectic is an inquiry into the principle "that the series of conditions . . . extends to the unconditioned," which asks, "Does it, or does it not, have objective applicability?" (*C.P.R.*, p. 307; Ak. A308=B365). On this subject, cf. *C.P.R.*, A321–32=B377–89.

10. Ibid., pp. 410–11; Ak. A447=B475 (my emphasis).

11. L. Brunschvicg, *Écrits philosophiques* (Paris: Presses Universitaires de France, 1951), 1:286.

12. *C.P.R.*, p. 413; Ak. A449=B477 (my emphasis).

13. *Proleg.*, p. 103; Ak. 4:363 (my emphasis).

14. *C.P.R.*, p. 413; Ak. A450=B478 (my emphasis).

15. Ibid., pp. 413–14; Ak. A450=B478. Cf. F. Alquié, *La critique kantienne de la métaphysique* (Paris: Presses Universitaires de France, 1968), p. 81 n. 1: "Observing that a beginning can be first with respect to causality without being first in respect to time, Kant, while reasoning within the perspective of the dogmatists, prepares the way to his own theory, which sees in free choice a choice not in time." We should keep this interesting comment in mind as we pursue the object of our inquiry.

16. *C.P.R.*, p. 424; Ak. A466=B494.

17. *Proleg.*, p. 81; Ak. 4:340.

18. *C.P.R.*, p. 423; Ak. A464=B492. Cf. *C.P.R.*, pp. 9, 532, 556, Ak. 4:xii, A643=B671, A680=B708.

19. Kant to Garve, September 21, 1798, Ak. 12:257–58. Cited by Alquié, *La critique kantienne de la métaphysique*, p. 72, n. 1; and by Philonenko, *L'oeuvre de Kant* (Paris: Vrin, 1969), 1:263.

20. *C.P.R.*, p. 470; Ak. A542=B570 (my emphasis).

21. Ibid., p. 466; Ak. A536=B564 (my emphasis).

22. Ibid., p. 467; Ak. A538=B566.

23. Ibid., p. 466; Ak. A536=B564.

24. Ibid., p. 470; Ak. A543=B571.

25. Ibid., p. 466; Ak. A536=B564.

26. Ibid., p. 439; Ak. A491=B519. Cf. ibid., p. 467; Ak. A537=B565: "Those who follow the common view [concerning the *absolute reality* of appearances] have *never* been able to reconcile nature and freedom [my emphasis]." Cf. *C.Pr.R.,* p. 98; Ak. 5:95: "If we still wish to *save* [freedom] [my emphasis]," we must distinguish between appearances and things-in-themselves. If we refuse to admit this distinction, then "freedom would have to be rejected as a void and impossible concept."

27. *C.P.R.,* p. 441; Ak. A494=B522.

28. Ibid., p. 514; Ak. A613=B641.

29. Ibid., p. 461; Ak. A528=B556. Cf. ibid., pp. 461–64; Ak. A528–32=B556–60. Cf. *C.Pr.R.,* pp. 98–99; Ak. 5:95–96.

30. Ibid., p. 462; Ak. A529=B557.

31. Cf. ibid., pp. 116, 194–98, 208–12, 236, 461–64; Ak. B110, A158–62=B197–202, A177–81=B218–24, A215=B262, A528–32=B556–60. Cf. *C.Pr.R.,* pp. 98–99, Ak. 5:95–96. See also G. Granel, *L'équivoque ontologique de la pensée kantienne* (Paris: Gallimard, 1970), pp. 155–71.

32. *C.P.R.,* p. 463; Ak. A530=B558; *C.Pr.R.,* p. 98; Ak. 5:95. Cf. the note added to the second edition of *C.P.R.,* pp. 196–97; Ak. B201–2:

All combination (*conjunctio*) is either composition (*compositio*) or connection (*nexus*). The former is the synthesis of the manifold where its constituents do not necessarily belong to one another. For example, the two triangles into which a square is divided by its diagonal do not necessarily belong to one another. Such also is the synthesis of the *homogeneous* in everything which can be *mathematically* treated. This synthesis can itself be divided into that of *aggregation* and that of *coalition,* the former applying to *extensive* and the latter to *intensive* qualities. The second mode of combination (*nexus*) is the synthesis of the manifold so far as its constituents *necessarily belong to one another,* as, for example, the accident to some substance, or the effect to the cause. It is therefore synthesis of that which, though *heterogeneous,* is yet represented as combined *a priori.* This combination, as not being arbitrary and as concerning the connection of the *existence* of the manifold, I entitle *dynamical.* Such connection can itself, in turn, be divided into the *physical* connection of the appearances with one another, and their *metaphysical* connection in the *a priori* faculty of knowledge.

Cf. the commentary on this text in J. Vuillemin, *Physique et métaphysique kantiennes* (Paris: Presses Universitaires de France, 1955), pp. 20–21: "Accident and substance, or effect and cause, do not enjoy the same relation of homogeneity as do two points in a line; but they are necessarily interdependent, and the abstraction which would separate them in thought would at the same time deprive them of any reality."

33. *C.P.R.*, p. 463; Ak. A539=B558–59 (my emphasis).

34. Ibid., p. 468; Ak. A539=B567. Cf. J. Lachelier, quoted in "Sur la théorie kantienne de la liberté," *Bulletin de la Société francaise de philosophie,* meeting of October 27, 1904 (Paris: Colin, 1905), p. 5: "For Kant the idea of the cause is twofold, and two different words are employed to express it. First there is the acting being who produces an event: the cause [*Ursache*]; then there is the action by which it produces it: the causality [*Kausalität*]."

35. *C.P.R.*, p. 467; Ak. A537=B565.

36. *Proleg.*, p. 84; Ak. 4:343: "But in the connection of cause and effect homogeneity may indeed likewise be found but is not necessary." Cf. *Progress,* p. 119; Ak. 20:292.

37. *C.P.R.*, p. 462; Ak. A530=B558. Cf. *C.Pr.R.*, pp. 98–99; Ak. 5:95–96.

38. *Proleg.*, p. 83; Ak. 4:343.

39. *C.P.R.*, p. 464; Ak. A532=B560. Cf. *Proleg.*, pp. 83–84; Ak. 4:343. Cf. *Progress,* p. 217; Ak. 20:291.

40. Cf. ibid. Cf. ibid., p. 464 n.

41. Ibid., p. 472; Ak. A546–47=B574–75. Cf. *Reflexionen zur Moralphilosophie,* n. 6860, Ak. 19:183, cited by R. Daval, *La métaphysique de Kant* (Paris: Presses Universitaires de France, 1968), p. 204: "Freedom, for man, is the apperception of himself as an intellectual being who acts." Cf. *C.F.J.,* p. 285; Ak. 5:435, where man is "the only natural being in which we can recognize, on the side of its peculiar constitution, a supersensible faculty [i.e., freedom]."

42. Ibid., p. 153; Ak. B132.

43. Ibid., p. 273; Ak. A256=B311–12.

44. *F.M.M.*, p. 71; Ak. 4:452: "For this reason a rational being must regard himself as intelligence (and not from the side of his lower powers), as belonging to the world of understanding and not to that of the senses." Cf. *C.P.R.*, p. 472; Ak. A546–47=B574–75. Cf. *C.Pr.R.*, pp. 49–50; Ak. 5:48–49.

45. *C.P.R.*, p. 472; Ak. A546=B574.

46. *F.M.M.*, p. 70; Ak. 4:451.

47. Cf. S. Körner, "Kant's Conception of Freedom," in *Proceedings of the British Academy* (London: Oxford University Press, 1967), 53:205: "I may indeed without contradiction assume that some aspects of myself are unknowable to me, but not that I can know these unknowable aspects."

48. Cf. *C.P.R.*, p. 472; Ak. A547=B575. Cf. *F.M.M.*, p. 70; Ak. 4:452.

49. *Proleg.*, p. 87; Ak. 4:346. The nature of these objective principles of reason will be determined further when we raise the question of practical freedom; for now it is enough to demonstrate that reason can exist at the point of origin of a series of events.

50. Ibid., p. 86.

51. Ibid.
52. Ibid., p. 86; Ak. 4:345.
53. *C.P.R.*, pp. 467 and 472; Ak. A537=B565, A546=B574.
54. *Proleg.*, p. 86; Ak. 4:345 (my emphasis).
55. Ibid. (my emphasis).
56. Ibid., p. 85; Ak. 4:344 n.
57. Ibid.
58. *C.P.R.*, p. 467; Ak. A537=B565 (my emphasis).
59. Ibid., p. 48; Ak. A561=B589.
60. *Proleg.*, p. 85; Ak. 4:344 n.
61. *C.P.R.*, p. 481; Ak. A561=B589.
62. *Proleg.*, p. 85; Ak. 4:344 n.
63. Delbos, *La philosophie pratique de Kant*, p. 203.
64. Cf. *C.P.R.*, p. 9; Ak. Axii.
65. This demand for the unconditioned characterizes *pure* reason, whether speculative or practical. Hence Paton is right to say that "Kant is consistent in ascribing to *pure* practical reason the Idea of an unconditioned good, the Idea of an unconditioned principle (or law), and the Idea of an unconditioned or categorical imperative" (H. J. Paton, *The Categorical Imperative*, 6th ed. [London: Hutchinson, 1967], p. 100).
66. *C.P.R.*, p. 24; Ak. Bxx.
67. *Progress*, p. 109; Ak. 20:287.
68. *C.P.R.*, p. 465; Ak. A533=B561.
69. There is a divergence of interpretations on this point. Cf. P. F. Strawson, who asserts,

It has nothing to do with the interests of theoretical reason. It has to do with the interests of "pure practical reason," i.e. of morality. Kant is anxious to show that the causal determination of every event by temporally antecedent conditions is not incompatible with the idea of certain events having another kind of cause which, as belonging to the noumenal sphere, is exempt from the condition of time and may be thought of as "acting" freely. Though we cannot understand this possibility, we cannot rule it out on the ground of determinism in Nature; and it is something which morality seems to demand, though we cannot claim theoretical knowledge of it on that account (P. F. Strawson, *The Bounds of Sense* [London: Methuen and Co., 1966], p. 213).

Cf. Strawson, *Bounds of Sense*, p. 215. According to Lewis White Beck, on the other hand, "The interest of speculative, and not merely of practical reason lies on the side of freedom" (L. W. Beck, *A Commentary on Kant's "Critique of Practical Reason"* [Chicago: University of Chicago Press, Phoenix Books, 1966], p. 185).
70. *C.P.R.*, p. 654; Ak. A798=B826. (We know that the Canon of Pure Reason constitutes the oldest part of the *Critique*.)

132

71. Ibid., pp. 429–30; Ak. A474–75=B502–3.
72. Ibid., pp. 424–25; Ak. A466–67=B494–95.
73. Cf. *C.Pr.R.*, p. 3; Ak. 5:3 (my emphasis). Cf. *C.P.R.*, p. 413; Ak. A450=B478.
74. *C.Pr.R.*, p. 7; Ak. 5:7.
75. *C.P.R.*, pp. 300, 394; Ak. A298=B354, A422=B449.
76. Ibid., p. 318; Ak. A327=B383.
77. Ibid., p. 434; Ak. A482=B510.
78. Ibid., pp. 307, 319; Ak. A309=B366, A327=B384.
79. Ibid., p. 450; Ak. A509=B537.
80. Ibid., p. 438; Ak. A489=B517.
81. Ibid., p. 411; Ak. A447=B475. We may well be astonished to see a philosopher of freedom tell us about the illusion of freedom. But is it not precisely in order to "save" freedom (*"retten,"* *C.Pr.R.*, p. 55; Ak. 5:54; *"gerettet,"* *Proleg.*, p. 87; Ak. 4:346) that Kant denounces this illusion? For Kant, it is crucial to illuminate the error of believing that we can establish the objective *theoretical* reality of freedom through the mediation of a concept of reason before establishing the objective *practical* reality of freedom attested by a fact of reason.
82. *F.M.M.*, pp. 74–75; Ak. 4:455 (my emphasis).
83. *C.Pr.R.*, p. 107; Ak. 5:103.
84. *C.F.J.*, p. 188; Ak. 5:343. Cf. *F.M.M.*, pp. 66–68; Ak. 4:448–49.
85. *C.P.R.*, p. 28; Ak. Bxxviii.
86. Ibid., p. 411; Ak. A447=B475.
87. *Proleg.*, p. 74; Ak. 4:333.
88. Ibid.; Ak. 4:332.
89. *C.P.R.*, p. 479; Ak. A557–58=B585–86.
90. Ibid., p. 10; Ak. Axiii.
91. Ibid., p. 27 n; Ak. Bxxvin.
92. Cf. *C.Pr.R.*, p. 3; Ak. 5:3. Cf. *C.P.R.*, p. 479; Ak. A558=B586.
93. "What is Orientation in Thinking?" trans. and ed. L. W. Beck, in *Kant's "Critique of Practical Reason" and Other Writings in Moral Philosophy* (Chicago: University of Chicago Press, 1949), p. 297; Ak. 8:137.
94. *C.P.R.*, p. 28; Ak. Bxxviii.
95. Ibid., pp. 295, 503 n; Ak. A291=B348, A596=B624n.
96. Cf. ibid., pp. 27 n, 478–79, 503, 503n; Ak. Bxxvin, A244–46, A557–58=B585–86, A596=B624. On the question of logical possibility and real possibility, cf. H. J. Paton, *Kant's Metaphysic of Experience*, 4th ed. (London: George Allen and Unwin, 1965), 1:66; 2:344, 346, 351. A concept is possible, that is, *logically* possible, when it is not self-contradictory. But it does not follow from that that its object is possible. The *real* possibility of the object must be known otherwise. To be able to grant real possibility to

an object, "something more" is required; "this something more need not, however, be sought in the theoretical sources of knowledge; it may lie in those that are practical" (*C.P.R.*, p. 27 n; Ak. Bxxvi n). The concept of a thing which is really possible had an *objective reality*, or an objective value. Strictly speaking, the real possibility is therefore the possibility of the object. But Kant does not always employ the terminology so rigorously, and he occasionally speaks of the (real) possibility of a concept (the concept of a possible object being itself a possible concept) and does not distinguish the real possibility of the concept from its objective reality. Cf. *C.P.R.*, pp. 27 n, 241; Ak. Bxxvi n, A222=B269.

97. *M.P.V.*, p. 39; Ak. 4:382. Cf. *C.P.R.*, p. 240; Ak. A220=B268: "It is, indeed, a necessary logical condition that a concept of the possible must not contain any contradiction; but this is not by any means sufficient to determine the objective reality of the concept, that is, the possibility of such an object as is thought through the concept." Cf. *C.P.R.*, pp. 262–63; Ak. A244=B302: "For to substitute the logical possibility of the *concept* (namely, that the concept does not contradict itself) for the transcendental possibility of *things* (namely, that an object corresponds to the concept) can deceive and leave satisfied only the simple-minded."

98. *C.Pr.R.*, p. 49; Ak. 5:48.

99. Ibid., p. 50; Ak. 5:48.

100. Ibid., p. 137; Ak. 5:132. Cf. ibid., p. 97; Ak. 5:94.

101. *C.F.J.*, p. 318; Ak. 5:453: "But to assume the possibility of a supersensible Being determined according to certain concepts would be a completely groundless supposition. For here none of the conditions requisite for cognition, as regards that in it which rests upon intuition, is given, and so the sole criterion of possibility remaining is the mere principle of contradiction (which can only prove the possibility of the thought, not of the object thought)." Cf. *C.P.R.*, pp. 613–14; Ak. A771–72=B799–800.

102. *C.P.R.*, p. 271; Ak. B310. Cf. p. 270; Ak. A254.

103. *C.F.J.*, p. 327; Ak. 5:467–68. Cf. *C.Pr.R.*, p. 49; Ak. 5:48.

104. *C.Pr.R.*, pp. 3, 7; Ak. 5:3, 7. Cf. *C.P.R.*, pp. 271–72; Ak. A254–55=B310–11.

105. *C.Pr.R.*, p. 3; Ak. 5:3.

106. *C.P.R.*, p. 109; Ak. A74=B100. Cf. *Logic*, pp. 114–15; Ak. 9:108.

107. Ibid., p. 292; Ak. A286–87=B343. "Possible" should be understood here as "really possible."

108. Ibid., p. 602; Ak. A753=B781. Cf. ibid., pp. 594–95; Ak. A741–42=B769–70. Cf. *Progress*, p. 123; Ak. 20:294. Cf. *C.Pr.R.*, p. 148; Ak. 5:142.

109. "What is Orientation in Thinking?" p. 300; Ak. 8:141.

110. *C.P.R.*, p. 11; Ak. Axv.

111. Ibid., pp. 614–15; Ak. A772=B800.

112. Ibid., p. 615; Ak. A773–74=B800–802.
113. Ibid., pp. 613, 616; Ak. A770=B798, A775=B803.
114. The etymology of the verb "to work" (*besogner*) bears witness to the close relation between "labor" (*le travail*) and "need" (*le besoin*). The human being labors because he is needy—because need rules him.
115. *C.P.R.*, pp. 617–18; Ak. A777=B805.
116. Ibid., p. 620; Ak. A781=B809.
117. Ibid., p. 532; Ak. A642–43=B670–71: "Everything that has its basis in the nature of our powers must be appropriate to, and consistent with, their right employment—if only we can guard against a certain misunderstanding and so can discover the proper direction of these powers. We are entitled, therefore, to suppose that transcendental ideas have their own good, proper, and therefore *immanent* use." Cf. *Nachlass* n. 5602, Ak. 18:247, cited by L. Guillermit, trans., First Introduction to the *Critique of Judgement* (Paris: Vrin, 1968, n. 42): "The employment of concepts of the understanding was immanent, the employment of Ideas as concepts of objects is transcendent; but as regulative principles for the completion and demarcation of our knowledge they are immanent in a critical fashion."
118. Ibid., p. 615; Ak. A773=B801 (my emphasis).
119. Ibid., p. 257; Ak. A235=B294.
120. Ibid., p. 320; Ak. A329=B385. Cf. E. Weil, *Problèmes kantiens* (Paris: Vrin, 1963), p. 21.
121. Ibid., p. 533; Ak. A644=B672. Cf. *C.Pr.R.*, p. 50; Ak. 5:48: The concept of freedom is a "regulative principle of reason."
122. Cf. ibid., pp. 547, 550; Ak. A666=B694, A671=B699.
123. Ibid., p. 551; Ak. A672=B700. Cf. Paton, *The Categorical Imperative*, p. 100: "The only use of the Idea of an absolute totality of causes is, for theoretical reasons, a purely *regulative* one—that is, it does not help us to know objects (and so it is not what Kant calls '*constitutive*'), but it encourages us, when we have discovered a cause, to seek for a further cause, and so on indefinitely."
124. Ibid., p. 559; Ak. A685=B713.
125. Cf. Philonenko, *L'oeuvre de Kant* 1:323–24: "The 'as if,' far from representing a mere negation or inadequacy and signifying only that reason has ceased to be proud, points to something more fundamental and more original: *the essence of reason as a faculty of problems and a capacity for work and adaptation.*"
126. *C.P.R.*, p. 320; Ak. A329=B385.
127. Ibid., p. 549; Ak. A669=B697.
128. Cf. ibid., pp. 324, 549–50; Ak. A336=B393, A669–70=B697–98.
129. *C.P.R.*, p. 549; Ak. A669=B697.
130. Ibid., p. 614; Ak. A771=B799. Cf. ibid., p. 550; Ak. A671=B699.
131. Ibid., p. 550; Ak. A671=B699.

132. Cf. Hans Vaihinger, *The Philosophy of "As If,"* trans. C. K. Ogden (New York: Harcourt, Brace & Company, 1925), pp. 294–95. Cf. Gilles Deleuze, *Différence et Répétition* (Paris: Presses Universitaires de France, 1968), pp. 219–20: "Kant loves to say that the Idea as problem has a value which is at once objective and indeterminate. Indeterminacy is no longer a mere imperfection in our knowledge, nor is it a lack in the object; it is a quite positive objective structure, already acting in our perception like a horizon, or an antechamber. The indeterminate object—the object as Idea— enables us to represent other objects (those of experience), to which it lends a maximum systematic unity."

Chapter Two

1. *C.P.R.,* p. 465; Ak. A534=B562.
2. Ibid., p. 634; Ak. A802=B830.
3. Ibid. Freedom confirms the practical employment of reason as a fact, but this incontestable fact is a fact of experience, not a fact of reason. Cf. M. Guerolt, *Annuaire du Collège de France* 1959–60: 243–44.
4. Several passages from the first *Critique* testify to the close connection Kant establishes between freedom and duty. Cf. *C.P.R.,* pp. 472–75; Ak. A547–50=B575–79: "That our reason has causality, or that we at least represent it to ourselves as having causality, is evident from the *imperatives* which in all matters of conduct we impose as rules upon our active powers" (p. 472). Cf. *Proleg.,* pp. 83–88; Ak. 4:343–47. As J. Lachelier observes,

For Kant the proof of our freedom results from the fact that we dictate our own conduct to ourselves. We tell ourselves that we ought to do something or that we should not have done something which we have done. Now it is apparent that the word *ought* [*devoir*] is taken in quite another sense than when we say that an event must happen [*doit arriver*] (that is, that it cannot not happen) by virtue of the causal connection of appearances: for the act that we ought to do is often an act that we do not do, and our obligation to do it does not proceed from a prior act (Lachelier, "Sur la théorie Kantienne de la liberté," pp. 5–6).

5. *Diss.,* p. 49 n; Ak. 2:396 n (my emphasis).
6. *C.P.R.,* p. 636; Ak. A807=B835 (my emphasis).
7. Ibid., p. 637; Ak. A807=B835.
8. Ibid., p. 632; Ak. A800=B828: "*Moral* laws . . . alone, therefore, belong to the practical employment of reason, and allow of a canon."
9. Ibid., p. 640; Ak. A813=B841 (my emphasis).
10. Ibid., p. 639; Ak. A811=B839.
11. Ibid., p. 473; Ak. A547–48=B575–76 (my emphasis).
12. Ibid.; Ak. A548=B576. Cf. M. Guerolt, "L'antidogmatisme de Kant et de Fichte," *Revue de métaphysique et de morale,* 1920, p. 189. Cf. Delbos, *La philosophie pratique de Kant,* p. 182.
13. *C.P.R.,* p. 634; Ak. A803=B831.

14. Ibid. Cf. Delbos, *La philosophie pratique de Kant*, pp. 191–92. Cf. M. Guerolt, "Canon de la raison pure et critique de la raison pratique," *Revue internationale de philosophie* 4 (1954): p. 338–40. Lewis White Beck does not share this interpretation:

> Section I of the Canon of Pure Reason is often regarded as having asserted that practical freedom is independent of transcendental freedom. . . . The last paragraph of Section I does not say that practical freedom could stand if transcendental freedom were not real; it says merely that this question does not concern us in the practical field or in a canon where we "demand of reason nothing but the rule of conduct. . . ." (*A Commentary on Kant's "Critique of Practical Reason,"* p. 190, n. 40).

15. Cf. Delbos, *La philosophie pratique de Kant*, p. 190, n. 2.

16. *C.P.R.*, p. 412; Ak. A448=B476.

17. Ibid., p. 465; Ak. A533=B561.

18. Ibid., p. 634; Ak. A803=B831 (my emphasis).

19. Ibid., p. 465; Ak. A534=B562.

20. Ibid. (my emphasis).

21. Ibid.

22. *Proleg.*, pp. 86–87; Ak. 4:346: "Freedom is therefore no hindrance to natural law in appearances; neither does this law abrogate the freedom of the practical use of reason, which is connected with things in themselves, as determining grounds. *Thus* practical freedom, viz., the freedom in which reason possesses causality according to objectively determining grounds, *is rescued;* and yet natural necessity is not in the least curtailed with regard to the very same effects, as appearances" (my emphasis).

23. *C.P.R.*, p. 634; Ak. A803=B831 (my emphasis).

24. Guerolt, "Canon de la raison pure et critique de la raison pratique," p. 340.

25. *C.P.R.*, p. 472; Ak. A547=B575.

26. Ibid., p. 473; Ak. A548–49=B576–77 (my emphasis).

Chapter Three

1. *C.P.R.*, p. 468; Ak. A539=B657.

2. Ibid., p. 472; Ak. A546=B574.

3. Ibid., pp. 472–73; Ak. A546–47=B574–75.

4. Ibid., p. 467; Ak. A538=B566.

5. Ibid., p. 468; Ak. A539=B567. Cf. *Anthropology*, p. 195; Ak. 7:285: "In pragmatic consideration, the universal, natural (not civil) signification of the word *character* is twofold; sometimes people say that a certain person has this or that character; and sometimes people say that a person has simply character (a moral character) which defines him as an individual and no one else. The first is man's mark of difference as a creature with senses or

a being of Nature; the second is the distinguishing mark of a reasonable being endowed with freedom." This passage clearly expresses the dual placement of character. Cf. L. Guillermit and J. Vuillemin, *Le Sens du destin* (Neuchâtel: Éditions de la Baconnière, 1948), p. 202.

6. Lachelier, "Sur la théorie kantienne de la liberté," p. 11.

7. *C.P.R.*, pp. 476–77; Ak. A553–54=B581–82.

8. Ibid., p. 472; Ak. A546=B574.

9. Ibid., pp. 468–69; Ak. A539–41=B567–69. Time is an a priori form of sensibility. It is "the formal . . . a priori condition of all appearance whatsoever" (*C.P.R.*, p. 77; Ak. A34=B50). In the Transcendental Aesthetic Kant's conception of time is confined to the time of representation; nevertheless, in other works it is enriched by a practical dimension. Cf. Paul Ricoeur, *The Conflict of Interpretations*, ed. Don Ihde (Evanston, Ill.: Northwestern University Press, 1974), pp. 416 ff.

10. J. Nabert, *L'expérience intérieure de la liberté* (Paris: Presses Universitaires de France, 1924), p. 152.

11. Guerolt, "L'antidogmatisme de Kant et de Fichte," p. 213.

12. Ibid., p. 214. J.-L. Bruch warns us, in the same way and for the same reasons, against a premature assimilation of the *status noumenon* to the permanent and immutable, for, he says, the latter are defined as a function of phenomenal time and thus have a purely phenomenal character themselves. "When one takes away from the thing-in-itself a phenomenal attribute—for example, phenomenal alteration—one does not thereby confer on it the opposite phenomenal attribute" (J.-L. Bruch, *La philosophie religieuse de Kant* [Paris: Aubier, 1968], p. 89).

13. *C.P.R.*, p. 478; Ak. A556=B584.

14. Ibid., p. 476; Ak. A553=B581 (my emphasis).

15. Ibid., p. 477; Ak. A555=B583.

16. Ibid., p. 467; Ak. A538=B566 (my emphasis).

17. Ibid., p. 476; Ak. A552=B580.

18. Ibid., p. 474; Ak. A549=B577.

19. Ibid.

20. Ibid., p. 472; Ak. A546=B574 (my emphasis).

21. Ibid., p. 478; Ak. A556=B584.

22. Cf. Lachelier, "Sur la théorie kantienne de la liberté," pp. 6–7: "Through the mediation of its maxims, our reason determines, *at least in part*, our empirical character." For his part, Norman Kemp Smith claims, "The *entire* empirical character is determined by the intelligible character" (Norman Kemp Smith, *A Commentary to Kant's "Critique of Pure Reason"* [New York: Humanities Press, 1962], p. 516).

23. *C.P.R.*, p. 476; Ak. A553=B581 (my emphasis). J. Lachelier notes that "the most difficult thing is to understand how this intelligible causality

determines our phenomenal causality and, through the mediation of the latter, modifies the course of events in the world" ("Sur la théorie kantienne de la liberté," p. 6).

24. Ibid., p. 467; Ak. A537=B565 (my emphasis). Do the negative definition and the positive definition of freedom correspond to empirical character and intelligible character respectively? Evidently this is Lewis White Beck's position when he writes, "The freedom of the empirical character is at first to be understood only negatively, as not being necessitated by things in nature. The freedom of the [intelligible character] is positive, for it originates a series of events in the world which would not have happened, had the intelligible character been different" (Beck, *A Commentary on Kant's "Critique of Practical Reason,"* p. 191). The passages in the first *Critique* on which he bases his claim (*C.P.R.*, p. 477; Ak. A554=B582) do not seem to us to justify such an interpretation. Further, Kant clearly affirms that "as regards this empirical character there is no freedom" (*C.P.R.*, p. 474; Ak. A550=B578). For us, the empirical character is only the appearance of intelligible character.

25. *C.P.R.*, p. 468; Ak. A540=B568. Cf. Daval, *La métaphysique de Kant,* pp. 214–16.

26. *C.P.R.*, p. 469; Ak. A541=B569.

27. Cf. J. Lachelier, *Oeuvres de Jules Lachelier* (Paris: Alcan, 1933), 2:210.

28. *C.P.R.*, p. 472; Ak. A546=B574 (my emphasis).

29. Ibid., p. 469; Ak. A541=B569 (my emphasis). Cf. *C.P.R.*, p. 473; Ak. A549=B577: "Reason . . . must . . . exhibit [*zeigen*] an empirical character."

30. Ibid., p. 181; Ak. A138=B177.

31. Ibid., p. 476; Ak. A553=B581 (my emphasis).

32. Ibid., p. 186; Ak. A146=B186.

33. Ibid., p. 468; Ak. A540=B568.

34. Ibid., p. 475; Ak. A551=B579.

35. Ibid., p. 475 n; Ak. A551=B579 n.

36. Cf. ibid., p. 412; Ak. A448=B476.

37. Ibid., p. 477; Ak. A555=B583. Cf. *Religion*, p. 33; Ak. 6:38.

38. *C.P.R.*, p. 477; Ak. A555=B583. Cf. Alquié, *La critique kantienne de la métaphysique*, p. 100: "The second *Critique* distinguishes two aspects of freedom. On one side, freedom, as autonomy, is revealed as identical to the law. On the other side, it appears as the source of our character, which can be wicked, and so contrary to the law. This distinction is latent in the text of the antinomy, where Kant first ties freedom to duty, and is then invoked again in the analysis of moral judgment based on fault."

39. *C.P.R.*, p. 477; Ak. A555=B583.

40. Ibid., p. 477; Ak. A554=B582 (my emphasis).

41. Ibid., p. 478; Ak. A557=B585 (my emphasis).
42. Ibid., p. 475 n; Ak. A551=B579 n.

Conclusion to Part I

1. *C.P.R.*, p. 46; Ak. B7. Cf. ibid., p. 325 n; Ak. B395 n. P. 631; Ak. A798=B826. Cf. *C.F.J.*, p. 325; Ak. 5:465.
2. Ibid., p. 7; Ak. Avii.
3. *F.M.M.*, p. 75; Ak. 4:456.
4. *C.P.R.*, p. 26; Ak. Bxxiv (my emphasis).
5. *Proleg.*, p. 85; Ak. 4:344.
6. *C.P.R.*, p. 28; Ak. Bxxviii.
7. Ibid., pp. 28–9; Ak. Bxxviii–xxix.
8. Ibid., p. 27; Ak. Bxxv. Cf. Granel, *L'équivoque ontologique*, p. 157:

The mathematical antinomies are both set aside as false (that is, as not signifying anything), while the dynamical antinomies escape to οὐδέν λέγειν. They are taken as genuinely *saying* something in both their theses and their antitheses in such a way that it is necessary to conceive as their subject a transaction between what each one signifies rather than simply their mutual effacement in meaninglessness. In this way the distinction of the mathematical and the dynamical assumes the magnitude of a decisive turning point in Kant's thought. If the language of freedom and causality in their antinomy had been shown to be as empty of meaning as that of the mathematical series in its, we would have had no means of getting to a practical reason whose very vocabulary had not been nullified instead of merely lacking completion through an intuition.

9. *C.P.R.*, pp. 313–14; Ak. A319=B375–76.
10. *F.M.M.*, p. 76; Ak. 4:456.
11. *Reflexionen zur Metaphysik*, Ak. 18:669, cited in G. Martin, *Science moderne et ontologie traditionnelle chez Kant*, trans. J.-C. Piguet (Paris: Presses Universitaires de France, 1963), p. 146. Not only does the ideality of space and time destroy the pretensions of speculative metaphysics, it is also the key to the solution of the antinomies and one of the principles which allow us to establish the logical possibility of freedom.

Chapter Four

1. *F.M.M.*, p. 18; Ak. 4:402.
2. Ibid., p. 39; Ak. 4:421 (my emphasis).
3. Cf. ibid., p. 37; Ak. 4:420.
4. Ibid., pp. 42–43; Ak. 4:425.
5. Ibid., p. 47; Ak. 4:428.
6. Paton, *The Categorical Imperative*, p. 129.
7. *F.M.M.*, p. 39; Ak. 4:421.
8. Ibid.
9. Ibid., p. 47; Ak. 4:429.

10. Ibid., p. 52; Ak. 4:434.

11. Ibid., p. 57; Ak. 4:438.

12. Ibid., p. 55; Ak. 4:437.

13. Ibid., p. 54; Ak. 4:436.

14. Ibid., p. 55; Ak. 4:436–37.

15. Ibid., p. 49; Ak. 4:431.

16. Ibid., p. 59; Ak. 4:440.

17. Ibid.

18. Ibid., p. 39; Ak. 4:421: "All the imperatives of duty can be derived from this one imperative as a principle."

19. Ibid., p. 55; Ak. 4:436.

20. Ibid., p. 49; Ak. 4:431 (my emphasis).

21. Ibid., p. 59; Ak. 4:440.

22. Ibid., p. 50; Ak. 4:431–32 (my emphasis).

23. Ibid., p. 51; Ak. 4:432–33. This is why the "pure moral law" of the Canon of Pure Reason cannot be considered absolutely pure. It is not presented in the form of a genuine categorical imperative; it carries an implicit interest, and it affects the subject's sensibility with "threats" and "promises." Cf. *C.P.R.*, p. 639; Ak. A811=B839.

24. *F.M.M.*, pp. 52–53; Ak. 4:434.

25. Ibid., p. 43; Ak. 4:425.

26. Ibid., p. 64; Ak. 4:445 (my emphasis).

27. Ibid. (my emphasis).

28. Ibid., p. 39; Ak. 4:421.

29. Kant's text indicates that for a holy will, the categorical imperative will be analytic (*F.M.M.*, p. 38n; Ak. 4:420n). Indeed, in such a case it would no longer concern a categorical imperative but rather the moral law of which the categorical imperative is only the expression for a will which is specifically not holy. This does not prevent Kant from asserting in the second *Critique* that the moral law is synthetic a priori (*C.Pr.R.*, p. 31; Ak. 5:31). Lewis White Beck maintains that this is a contradiction in his article "Apodictic Imperatives" (*Kantstudien* 49 [1957]: 12n [reproduced in L. W. Beck, *Studies in the Philosophy of Kant* (New York: Liberal Arts Press, 1965), pp. 177–99]). In fact, as B. Rousset observes, "the context shows that it is not the presence of the law but its existence for us in the form of duty which is synthetic" (B. Rousset, *La doctrine kantienne de l'objectivité* [Paris: Vrin, 1967], p. 529 n. 26).

30. *F.M.M.*, p. 38, 38n; Ak. 4:420, 420n.

31. *C.Pr.R.*, p. 31; Ak. 5:31. This expression is not to be found in the *Grundlegung.*

32. *F.M.M.*, p. 64; Ak. 4:446.

33. Ibid.

34. Ibid., p. 29; Ak. 4:412.

35. Cf. *C.P.R.*, pp. 410–11; Ak. A447=B475.

36. *F.M.M.*, p. 65; Ak. 4:446–47.

37. Kant expresses this double opposition in a particularly felicitous formula when he defines practical freedom as "the will's independence of everything except the moral law" (*C.Pr.R.*, p. 97; Ak. 5:94).

38. *F.M.M.*, p. 65; Ak. 4:447. Cf. *C.Pr.R.*, p. 47; Ak. 5:46: "If the will is presupposed as free, then [practical laws] are necessary."

39. *C.Pr.R.*, p. 31; Ak. 5:31. Cf. *C.Pr.R.*, p. 97; Ak. 5:93–94: "If we saw the possibility of freedom of an efficient cause, we would see not only the possibility but also the necessity of the moral law as the supreme practical law of rational beings. . . . But the possibility of freedom of an efficient cause cannot be comprehended, especially in the world of sense."

40. *F.M.M.*, p. 65; Ak. 4:447.

41. Ibid., p. 72; Ak. 4:453.

42. Ibid. Cf. ibid., p. 69; Ak. 4:451.

43. Ibid. Cf. *M.P.R.*, p. 21; Ak. 6:221: "Upon this [positive] concept of freedom . . . are founded unconditional practical laws, which are called moral."

44. *F.M.M.*, p. 73; Ak. 4:454 (my emphasis).

45. Ibid., p. 72; Ak. 4:453.

46. Ibid., p. 71; Ak. 4:452 (my emphasis).

47. *C.Pr.R.*, p. 47; Ak. 5:46.

48. Ibid., p. 100; Ak. 5:97 (my emphasis). Cf. ibid., p. 99; Ak. 5:96: The question of freedom "lies at the foundation of all moral laws and accountability [*Zurechnung*] to them."

49. *Recension von Schulz's Versuch einer Anleitung zur Sittenlehre für alle Menschen*, Ak. 8:13, cited by Delbos, *La philosophie pratique de Kant*, p. 218.

50. Cf. *C.F.J.*, p. 323; Ak. 5:471 n.

51. *C.Pr.R.*, p. 4 n; Ak. 5:4 n.

52. Ibid., p. 4; Ak. 5:4.

53. *C.P.R.*, pp. 28–29; Ak. Bxxviii–xxix.

54. "What is Orientation in Thinking?" p. 298; Ak. 8:139. (Written in 1786.)

55. Philonenko, *L'oeuvre de Kant* 1:333–34: "The moral problem was not developed at length in the first *Critique*. Of course, Kant was able to recast the second edition on this point—but was this really needed? At the same time that Kant, on the invitation of his editor Hartknoch, revised the first *Critique*, the second *Critique* was already on its way to the printer."

56. *C.Pr.R.*, p. 29; Ak. 5:29–30.

57. Ibid., p. 31; Ak. 5:31.

58. Ibid., p. 48; Ak. 5:47. Cf. ibid., pp. 31, 43; Ak. 5:31, 42.

59. Ibid., p. 31; Ak. 5:31.

60. Ibid., p. 48; Ak. 5:47.

61. Ibid. Cf. ibid., pp. 57, 94, 108; Ak. 5:55, 91, 104.

62. Reason, G. Krüger says, endeavors to find authentic principles. But it seeks its independence where it cannot possibly find it: in the act of theoretical understanding. This is the danger to which the critique responds— a danger which the logic had already indicated: "The term 'principle' is ambiguous, and commonly signifies any knowledge which can be used as a principle [*als Prinzip*], although in itself, and as regards its proper origin, it is not principle [*principium*]. Every universal proposition, even one derived from experience, through induction, can serve as major premise in a syllogism; but it is not therefore itself a principle" (*C.P.R.*, p. 301; Ak. A300=B356). In morals, an authentic principle, in the form of a fact of reason, is *given* to the finite man. Cf. G. Krüger, *Critique et morale chez Kant*, trans. M. Régnier (Paris: Beauchesne, 1961), p. 41.

63. *C.Pr.R.*, p. 31; Ak. 5:31 (my emphasis).

64. Ibid., pp. 48, 94; Ak. 5:47, 91.

65. Ibid., p. 57; Ak. 5:55. Cf. Krüger, *Critique et morale chez Kant*, p. 227.

66. Cf. *Von einem neuerdings erhobenen vornehmen Ton in der Philosophie*, Ak. 8:402.

67. *C.Pr.R.*, p. 47; Ak. 5:46 (my emphasis). Cf. *M.P.R.*, p. 25; Ak. 6:225: "Practical laws . . . , like mathematical postulates, [are] indemonstrable and yet apodictic." Cf. *C.F.J.*, p. 322; Ak. 5:470: "If the supreme principle of all moral laws is a postulate, so is also the possibility of its highest object, and consequently, too, the condition under which we can think this possibility is postulated along with it and by it." Elsewhere, Kant asserts that "the principle of morality . . . is not a postulate but a law" (*C.Pr.R.*, p. 137; Ak. 5:132).

68. *C.Pr.R.*, p. 48; Ak. 5:47.

69. *Opus Postumum*, Ak. 21:421 (my emphasis).

70. *Religion*, p. 21; Ak. 6:26.

71. *Logic*, p. 98; Ak. 9:93.

72. *C.Pr.R.*, p. 48; Ak. 5:47.

73. Ibid., p. 49; Ak. 5:47.

74. Ibid. Evidently Kant, in the period 1776–78, did not consider that only the consciousness of the moral law could reveal the existence of freedom to us. "Transcendental freedom," he claims, "is the characteristic of beings for whom the consciousness of a rule is the basis of actions" (*Reflexionen zur Metaphysik* n. 4904, Ak. 18:24). The mere consciousness of a faculty, not necessarily moral, of accepting or refusing rules or principles can be interpreted as the *ratio cognoscendi* of freedom. Cf. Körner, "Kant's Conception of Freedom," p. 203.

75. *Opus Postumum,* Ak. 21 : 19 (my emphasis).
76. Ibid., Ak. 21 : 16.
77. Cf. *C.Pr.R.,* pp. 31, 165; Ak. 5:31, 161. Cf. *Religion,* pp. 40, 45 n, 46; Ak. 6:45, 49 n, 50. Cf. *Theory-Practice,* pp. 54–55; Ak. 8:287–88. Cf. *Confl. Fac.,* pp. 75–77; Ak. 7:43–44. On this point, cf. also the analysis by Rousset, *La doctrine kantienne,* p. 533.
78. *Progress,* p. 157; Ak. 20:311.
79. *Reflexionen zur Metaphysik* n. 6344, Ak. 18:669.
80. *C.Pr.R.,* p. 6; Ak. 5:6.
81. *Opus Postumum,* Ak. 21 : 16 (my emphasis).
82. *Recension von Schulz's Versuch,* Ak. 8 : 13.
83. Rousset, *La doctrine kantienne,* p. 534.
84. *C.P.R.,* p. 25; Ak. Bxxi. Cf. P. Burgelin, "Kant et les fins de la raison," *Revue de métaphysique et de morale* 58 (1953), p. 151. Cf. *C.Pr.R.,* p. 18; Ak. 5:20: Practical philosophy "has to do only with the grounds of determination of the will."
85. *C.Pr.R.,* p. 51; Ak. 5:50.
86. Ibid., p. 109; Ak. 5:105.
87. Ibid., p. 57; Ak. 5:55. Cf. ibid., p. 4; Ak. 5:4–5.
88. Cf. ibid., p. 58; Ak. 5:56. Cf. ibid., p. 49; Ak. 5:48. Cf. *C.P.R.,* p. 27 n; Ak. Bxxvi n. Cf. *C.Pr.R.,* pp. 58–59; Ak. 5:58.
89. *C.Pr.R.,* p. 4; Ak. 5:4.
90. Ibid., p. 49; Ak. 5:47.
91. Ibid., p. 49; Ak. 5:48. Cf. *M.P.R.,* p. 26; Ak. 6:226: "Freedom . . . first [*allererst*] becomes known to us through the moral law."
92. *C.Pr.R.,* p. 97; Ak. 5:94.
93. Ibid., p. 30; Ak. 5:30.
94. Ibid., p. 4 n; Ak. 5:4.
95. To allege that this is a vicious circle would be to forget that the distinction between the levels of being and of knowing is well established and testifies to the finitude of the mind. Kant clearly foresaw this objection. Cf. *F.M.M.,* pp. 68–69; Ak. 4:450; *C.Pr.R.,* p. 4 n; Ak. 5:4 n.
96. *C.Pr.R.,* p. 50; Ak. 5:49.
97. Ibid., p. 31; Ak. 5:31 (my emphasis).
98. Ibid., p. 97; Ak. 5:93.
99. Ibid., p. 48; Ak. 5:47.
100. Ibid., p. 97; Ak. 5:93 (my emphasis).
101. Ibid., p. 97; Ak. 5:94. Cf. ibid., p. 4; Ak. 5:4.
102. Cf. ibid., pp. 3, 7; Ak. 5:3, 7. Cf. ibid., pp. 49–50; Ak. 5:48. Cf. ibid., p. 5; Ak. 5:5. It is true that by proving the reality of freedom the moral law satisfied the *need* of theoretical reason, even while involving it in the greatest *difficulties.* Thus it will not surprise us that the *Critique of Pure*

Reason did not familiarize us with theoretical reason's ambivalence toward freedom, an ambivalence which is interpreted as a conflict of reason with itself. The solution of the third antinomy indicated how this conflict—this ambivalence—could be overcome.

103. *C.Pr.R.,* p. 49; Ak. 5:47.

104. Ibid., pp. 48–49; Ak. 5:47–48.

105. Cf. ibid., p. 7; Ak. 5:7.

106. Delbos, *La philosophie pratique de Kant,* p. 357.

107. *C.P.R.,* p. 25; Ak. Bxxi (my emphasis).

108. *C.Pr.R.,* p. 3; Ak. 5:3. The concepts of pure practical reason, notably the concept of freedom, are not "like the props and buttresses which usually have to be put behind a hastily erected building, but they are rather true members making the structure of the system plain and letting the concepts, which were previously [in the first *Critique*] thought of only in a problematic way, be clearly seen as real" (*C.Pr.R.,* p. 7; Ak. 5:7).

109. Ibid., p. 29; Ak. 5:29.

110. *Opus Postumum,* Ak. 21:30. Cf. *O.P.,* Ak. 21:16, 22:53.

111. *C.Pr.R.,* p. 29; Ak. 5:30 (my emphasis).

112. Ibid., p. 30; Ak. 5:30.

113. Ibid.

114. Ibid., p. 31; Ak. 5:31.

115. Ibid., p. 97; Ak. 5:93.

116. *F.M.M.,* p. 69; Ak. 4:450.

117. *C.Pr.R.,* p. 43; Ak. 5:42 (my emphasis).

118. Ibid., p. 43; Ak. 5:41–42 (my emphasis).

119. Ibid., p. 57; Ak. 5:55 (my emphasis). Cf. *Opus Postumum,* Ak. 21:421: "The moral law imposes itself here as an axiom and *contains* that causality in its own term" (my emphasis).

120. *C.Pr.R.,* p. 31; Ak. 5:31 (my emphasis).

121. Ibid., p. 57; Ak. 5:55.

122. Cf. the interpretation of Krüger, *Critique et morale chez Kant,* pp. 226–34.

123. Fichte, *System der Sittenlehre nach den Prinzipien der Wissenschaftslehre* (Meiner, 1969), p. 144, cited by Guerolt, "L'antidogmatisme de Kant et de Fichte," p. 192. On Fichte's critique of Kant on the subject of the "sole fact of reason," cf. Philonenko, *La liberté humaine dans la philosophie de Fichte* (Paris: Vrin, 1966), p. 60. Cf. Philonenko, *Théorie et praxis,* p. 160, n. 41.

124. *C.Pr.R.,* p. 30; Ak. 5:30.

125. *C.F.J.,* p. 321; Ak. 5:468.

126. Ibid., p. 326; Ak. 5:474.

127. *F.M.M.,* p. 74; Ak. 4:455.

128. *Logic,* p. 97; Ak. 9:92.

129. *F.M.M.*, p. 66; Ak. 4:447–48.

130. *C.Pr.R.*, p. 29; Ak. 5:29.

131. *C.F.J.*, p. 321; Ak. 5:468.

132. Ibid., p. 327; Ak. 5:474 (my emphasis).

133. Ibid., p. 321; Ak. 5:468 (my emphasis). Cf. Guerolt, "L'antidogmatisme de Kant et de Fichte," p. 188 n: "The experience of actions by itself would be incapable of showing the reality of freedom were there not a priori practical laws of reason, in conformity with which these actions happen."

134. *Opus Postumum*, Ak. 21:51–52. Cf. on this subject J. Lacroix, *Kant et le Kantisme* (Paris: Presses Universitaires de France, 1966), pp. 97–98.

135. *Verkündigung des nahen Abschlusses: eines Tractats zum ewigen Frieden in der Philosophie*, Ak. 8:416.

136. *C.Pr.R.*, pp. 108–9; Ak. 5:104–5.

137. Ibid., p. 48; Ak. 5:47.

138. Ibid., p. 43; Ak. 5:42 (my emphasis).

139. Perhaps Kant here rediscovers an idea of which he was already fond and which he had affirmed many times before: "Every being which cannot act otherwise than under the idea of freedom is thereby really free in a practical respect" (*F.M.M.*, p. 66; Ak. 4:448). "Man acts according to the idea of freedom, he acts *as if* he were free, and *eo ipso* he is free" (*Lectures on Philosophical Theology*, trans. Allen W. Wood and Gertrude M. Clark [Ithaca: Cornell University Press, 1978], p. 105, cited by Delbos, *La philosophie pratique de Kant*, p. 213).

140. *C.Pr.R.*, p. 109; Ak. 5:105.

141. Ibid., p. 4; Ak. 5:4.

142. *C.F.J.*, p. 327; Ak. 5:474.

143. Ibid., p. 321; Ak. 5:468.

144. *C.Pr.R.*, p. 4; Ak. 5:4 (my emphasis). This question will be taken up again and approached from another angle when we analyze the postulate of freedom.

145. Ibid., p. 107; Ak. 5:103.

146. *C.P.R.*, p. 25; Ak. Bxxi.

147. *C.Pr.R.*, p. 107; Ak. 5:103 (my emphasis).

148. Ibid., p. 117; Ak. 5:113.

149. Ibid., pp. 3–4; Ak. 5:3–4 (my emphasis).

150. *C.F.J.*, pp. 326–27; Ak. 5:474.

151. *C.Pr.R.*, p. 4; Ak. 5:4.

152. *C.F.J.*, p. 327; Ak. 5:474. Cf. *Progress*, p. 125; Ak. 20:295.

153. *C.F.J.*, p. 327; Ak. 5:474.

154. *Progress*, p. 125; Ak. 20:295.

155. *C.Pr.R.*, p. 109; Ak. 5:105 (my emphasis).

156. *C.F.J.*, pp. 12, 321; Ak. 5:176, 469.

157. Ibid., p. 322; Ak. 5:470 (my emphasis).

158. Ibid., pp. 326–27; Ak. 5:474: "Here the supersensible (freedom), which in this case is fundamental, . . . establishes its reality in actions as a fact."

159. Ibid., p. 326; Ak. 5:473–74 (my emphasis).

160. *C.Pr.R.*, p. 73; Ak. 5:70 (my emphasis).

161. *Logic*, p. 98; Ak. 9:93 (my emphasis). Placing these passages in context is enough to persuade us again that Kant in no way meant to reserve objective practical reality for the mere idea of freedom. This is why, immediately following the passage just cited, Kant adds, "The reality of the idea of God can be proved only through the moral law and therefore only with practical intent, i.e., the intent so to act as if there be a God—and this idea thus can be proved only for this intent" (p. 98; Ak. 9:93).

162. Cf. *C.Pr.R.*, pp. 5, 48, 49; Ak. 5:5, 47, 48. Cf. *Proleg.*, p. 84; Ak. 4:343: "But if natural necessity is referred merely to appearances and freedom merely to things in themselves, no contradiction arises if we at the same time assume or admit both kinds of causality, *however difficult or impossible* it may be to make the latter kind conceivable" (my emphasis).

163. *C.Pr.R.*, p. 97; Ak. 5:94.

164. *M.P.V.*, p. 37 n; Ak. 6:380n. Cf. *M.P.V.*, p. 78; Ak. 6:418.

165. *Religion*, p. 129; Ak. 6:138: "The ground [of freedom], inscrutable to us, . . . is a mystery because this ground is *not given* us as an object of knowledge."

166. *Religion*, p. 135 n. 2 (added in the second edition); Ak. 6:144n. Cf. O. Reboul, *Kant et le problème du mal* (Montréal: Presses de l'Université de Montréal, 1971), p. 162: "Such an admission cannot place the underlying unity of Kant's philosophy in doubt. For freedom, the central fact of the critical system, remains inexplicable—as a *fact* [*fait*]. It is absolutely clear that it is a possibility given to man from the moral law; but the real use man *makes* [*fait*] of this possibility remains incomprehensible to us."

167. *C.Pr.R.*, p. 50; Ak. 5:48. Cf. ibid., p. 57; Ak. 5:56: "Through [the *causa noumenon*] I do not strive to know theoretically the characteristic of a being in so far as it has a pure will."

168. *F.M.M.*, p. 78; Ak. 4:459.

169. *C.Pr.R.*, p. 75; Ak. 5:72: "For how a law in itself can be the direct determining ground of the will (which is the essence of morality) is an insoluble problem for the human reason. It is identical with the problem of how a free will is possible." Cf. *F.M.M.*, p. 80; Ak. 4:461.

170. *C.Pr.R.*, p. 47; Ak. 5:46: "How this consciousness of the moral laws or—what amounts to the same thing—how this consciousness of freedom is possible cannot be further explained [*weiter erklären*]."

171. *F.M.M.*, p. 80; Ak. 4:461.

172. Ibid., p. 80; Ak. 4:460.

173. Ibid., p. 64; Ak. 4:446.

174. Ibid., p. 65; Ak. 4:446.

175. *F.M.M.*, p. 31; Ak. 4:414.

176. M. Guerolt, *L'évolution et la structure de la doctrine de la science chez Fichte* (Paris: Les Belles Lettres, 1930), 1:42.

177. Cf. *F.M.M.*, p. 51; Ak. 4:433.

178. Martin Heidegger, *Kant and the Problem of Metaphysics*, trans. James S. Churchill (Bloomington: Indiana University Press, 1962), p. 165 (my emphasis).

179. Krüger, *Critique et morale chez Kant*, p. 94 n.

180. *C.Pr.R.*, p. 166; Ak. 5:161–62.

181. *Religion*, p. 21 n; Ak. 6:26 n.

182. *C.Pr.R.*, p. 109; Ak. 5:105 (my emphasis).

183. Ibid., p. 32; Ak. 5:32.

184. *F.M.M.*, p. 29; Ak. 4:412.

185. *C.Pr.R.*, p. 45; Ak. 5:44 (my emphasis).

186. Ibid., p. 166; Ak. 5:161–62. Cf. ibid., p. 32; Ak. 5:32: "Now this principle of morality, on account of the universality of its legislation which makes it the formal supreme determining ground of the will regardless of any subjective differences among men, is *declared* by reason to be a *law for all rational beings* in so far as they have a will, i.e., faculty of determining their causality through the conception of a rule." (my emphasis).

187. *F.M.M.*, pp. 73–74; Ak. 4:454–55. Cf. *M.P.V.*, p. 36; Ak. 6:379: "Men as rational natural beings . . . are unholy enough to be influenced by pleasure to transgress the moral law, although they recognize its authority." Cf. *Religion*, p. 31; Ak. 6:36.

188. *C.Pr.R.*, pp. 109–10; Ak. 5:105–6.

189. *Education*, p. 112; Ak. 9:494. Cf. *M.P.R.*, p. 27; Ak. 6:227: "He who commands (*imperans*) by a law is the lawgiver (*legislator*). He is the author (*auctor*) of the obligation imposed by the law but is not always the author of the law."

190. *C.Pr.R.*, p. 31; Ak. 5:31 (my emphasis).

191. *F.M.M.*, p. 52; Ak. 4:434 (my emphasis).

192. *C.Pr.R.*, p. 89; Ak. 5:87.

193. Ibid., p. 32; Ak. 5:32.

194. Ibid., p. 101; Ak. 5:97 (my emphasis). The reflexive verb indicates clearly that the action originates with the subject. Nevertheless, D. Julia believes it can be claimed that "the third maxim indicates that man is ordered [*a la consigne*] to think the law as if he himself were the creator of it. The *as if* literally means that man is the creator of the law, and that he

receives it passively" (D. Julia, *La question de l'homme et le fondement de la philosophie* [Paris: Aubier, 1964], p. 79). This does not seem to us a strict enough interpretation. First, the third formula of the imperative is an objective principle of action, not a maxim. Second, for man to consider himself the author of the law is not a moral duty but an absolute necessity arising from his nature as a rational being and concomitant with his freedom. This is Kant's meaning when he asserts that "the will of a rational being must always be considered as legislative" (*F.M.M.*, p. 52; Ak. 4:434), hence the use of the word "ordered" seems particularly unfortunate. Third, in using the expression "as if," Julia appeals less to the text itself than Krüger's interpretation of it (*Critique et morale chez Kant*, p. 129), for to our knowledge the expression *als ob* cannot be found in those passages where Kant talks about the third formula of the imperative (cf. *F.M.M.*, pp. 49, 52; Ak. 4:431, 434).

195. *F.M.M.*, pp. 51, 71; Ak. 4:433, 452.

196. *M.P.V.*, p. 101n; Ak. 6:439n. Cf. *M.P.R.*, p. 23; Ak. 6:223.

197. Cf. *F.M.M.*, p. 51; Ak. 4:433.

198. *F.M.M.*, p. 49; Ak. 4:431.

199. Ibid., p. 96; Ak. 4:440 (my emphasis).

200. Cf. *C.Pr.R.*, p. 28; Ak. 5:28–29. Cf. Guerolt, "L'antidogmatisme de Kant et de Fichte," p. 198: "The necessity with which reason lays down its law does not fatally suppress the genuine freedom of the act by which it does so, for reason lays it down by necessity only if and because it is free."

201. *M.P.R.*, p. 26; Ak. 6:226.

202. Ibid.

203. *F.M.M.*, p. 62; Ak. 4:443 (my emphasis). According to Weil's compelling observation, "morality must remain the morality of freedom; a morality imposed by an external authority would be immoral" (Weil, *Problèmes kantiens*, p. 94).

204. *C.Pr.R.*, p. 130; Ak. 5:125.

205. Ibid., p. 130; Ak. 5:125–26 (my emphasis).

206. Ibid., p. 152; Ak. 5:147. Cf. *C.F.J.*, pp. 311–12; Ak. 5:459–60. Cf. K. Jaspers, "Le mal radical chez Kant," *Deucalion* 4, no. 36 (1952): 247: "That a transcendent being is inaccessible to any knowledge, or experience, or any complete cognition, or subjective impression, or mystical apprehension—that is like a language of divinity, but an indirect language. If we could have such knowledge, our freedom would be paralyzed. Everything is as if the divinity willed to create the highest possible thing for us—the existence of freedom for its own sake—but that for this to be possible he was forced to hide himself." Cf. Weil, *Problèmes kantiens*, p. 68: "Kant wants as much to avoid all fatalistic determinism as he does a divine master, em-

pirically present to man, whose *known* power would render impossible every free decision, since freedom means something proceeding, not from fear, but from pure respect for the law that freedom gives itself" (Cf. Weil, *Problèmes kantiens,* pp. 44, 94).

207. *C.Pr.R.,* p. 32; Ak. 5 : 32.

208. Ibid. Cf. *F.M.M.,* pp. 29–30, 58; Ak. 4 : 413, 439.

209. *F.M.M.,* pp. 58, 51; Ak. 4 : 439, 414.

210. Heidegger, *Kant and Metaphysics,* p. 162.

211. *C.Pr.R.,* p. 83; Ak. 5 : 80.

212. Cf. ibid., p. 30; Ak. 5 : 30. Cf. *C.F.J.,* p. 319; Ak. 5 : 467.

213. *F.M.M.,* p. 16; Ak. 4 : 400.

214. Ibid. Cf. Paul Ricoeur, *Fallible Man,* trans. Charles Kelbley (Chicago: Henry Regnery, 1965).

215. *M.P.R.,* p. 21; Ak. 6 : 221.

216. *C.Pr.R.,* p. 97; Ak. 5 : 94 (my emphasis).

217. Ibid., p. 34; Ak. 5 : 33 (my emphasis).

218. *M.P.R.,* pp. 21–22; Ak. 6 : 222: "An imperative is a practical rule by which an action, in itself contingent, is made necessary. An imperative is distinguished from a practical law by the fact that while the latter represents the necessity of an action, it does not consider whether this necessity already resides by internal necessity in the acting subject (as in the case of a holy being), or whether, as in man, it is contingent; for where the internal necessity is the case, there is no imperative."

219. *F.M.M.,* p. 59; Ak. 4 : 440.

220. G. F. W. Hegel, *Philosophy of Right,* trans. T. M. Knox (London: Oxford University Press, 1952), p. 32.

221. *M.P.V.,* p. 101 n; Ak. 6 : 439 n.

222. Cf. ibid., pp. 36–40; Ak. 6 : 379–82.

223. Jean-Jacques Rousseau, *On the Social Contract,* trans. Judith R. Masters (New York: St. Martin's Press, 1978), p. 56

224. *F.M.M.,* p. 58; Ak. 4 : 439. Cf. *F.M.M.,* pp. 30–31; Ak. 4 : 413–14.

225. Ibid., p. 56; Ak. 4 : 437.

226. Ibid., p. 58; Ak. 4 : 440.

227. Ibid., p. 65; Ak. 4 : 447.

228. *M.P.V.,* p. 39 n; Ak. 6 : 382 n.

229. Heidegger, *Kant and Metaphysics,* p. 165.

230. Cf. *F.M.M.,* pp. 49, 58; Ak. 4 : 431, 440.

231. Cf. *C.F.J.,* p. 299 n; Ak. 5 : 448 n. On this point, see Paton, *The Categorical Imperative,* pp. 213–14.

232. *F.M.M.,* p. 74; Ak. 4 : 455.

233. Ibid., p. 42; Ak. 4 : 424.

234. *M.P.V.,* pp. 36–37 n; Ak. 6 : 380 n.

235. *C.Pr.R.,* p. 99; Ak. 5:96 (my emphasis).

236. *Religion,* p. 40; Ak. 6:44.

Chapter Five

1. Delbos and, following him, Lacroix both speak of "the act by which my will conforms itself to the law or places itself in rebellion against it" (V. Delbos, *Bulletin de la Sociéte francaise de philosophie,* p. 12; Lacroix, *Kant et le Kantisme,* p. 74). The term "rebellion" does not seem to express Kant's thought exactly. In transgressing the moral law, the human being does not act in a pure spirit of revolt; instead, he only subordinates the law to motives of sensibility. "Man (even the most wicked) does not, under any maxim whatsoever, repudiate the moral law in the manner of a rebel [*gleichsam rebellischerweise*] (renouncing obedience to it)" (*Religion,* p. 31; Ak. 6:36).

2. This is apparent notably in the second *Critique,* where Kant develops, first, the autonomy of the will (in the Analytic), second, freedom of choice (in the Critical Elucidation), and third, freedom as a postulate (in the Dialectic). Cf. the interesting observations of F. Alquié, *La morale de Kant* (Paris: Centre de documentation universitaire, 1959), pp. 96–100.

3. In the *Grundlegung, Wille* designates both autonomous will and free choice. Starting with the second *Critique,* however, the will endowed with free choice is more and more frequently called *Willkür,* the term Kant will employ almost constantly in the *Religion.* But it sometimes happens that we find *Willkür* where we would expect to see *Wille,* and vice versa. Cf. Delbos, *La philosophie pratique de Kant,* pp. 351 n. 2, 491 n. 1. [Kant's vocabulary of the will raises difficulties for the English translator, since there are no ready counterparts which consistently capture the contrast Kant developed between *Wille* and *Willkür.* This accounts for devices like the superscript " Theodore M. Greene and Hoyt H. Hudson used in their translation of Kant's *Religion* to indicate when the English "will" or "choice" translated *Willkür* rather than *Wille.* Of course the problem is compounded by the addition of a third vocabulary of the will, as in the present work. The French offers at least three alternatives to designate the legislative and elective functions of the will: *volonté, arbitre,* and *choix.* As a general rule, the author employs *volonté* for *Wille* and *choix* for *Willkür,* with *arbitre* rendering sometimes one, sometimes the other. Where possible we have relied on "will" when the author had Kant's *Wille* in mind, and "choice" when he had Kant's *Willkür* in mind. Following the author's suggestion, we have also sometimes employed the phrases "legislative will" to render *volonté* and "elective will" to render *arbitre* or *choix* when the intent was to contrast *Wille* and *Willkür.* When the context seemed to require "will" for *arbitre* when *Willkür* was intended, we have noted the exception in brackets or parentheses.—TRANS.]

4. *M.P.R.*, p. 26; Ak. 6:226.

5. Delbos claims that, in the *Religion*, "*Willkür* plainly names another type of will than that which lays down the moral law" (*La philosophie pratique de Kant*, p. 491 n. 1). We prefer to speak of two aspects of the will rather than of two types of will. Cf. Lewis White Beck's helpful comment in Beck, *A Commentary on Kant's "Critique of Practical Reason,"* pp. 198–99, 201.

6. We use here the terminology adopted by Paul Ricoeur. Cf. Ricoeur, *Conflict of Interpretations*, pp. 434, 438. In the same way, by translating *Willkür* as "elective will" and *Wille* as "will" or "rational will," T. K. Abbot enables us to avoid the error of opposing will and free choice; however, the expression "rational will" could easily let us suppose that the *Willkür* is not rational, when in reality it must be said that the *Willkür*, unlike the *Wille*, is not exclusively rational.

7. *C.Pr.R.*, p. 9n; Ak. 5:9n. Cf. *C.F.J.*, p. 14; Ak. 5:xxiiin. Cf. *M.P.R.*, p. 9; Ak. 6:211.

8. *M.P.R.*, p. 11; Ak. 6:213.

9. Ibid.

10. Ibid., p. 26; Ak. 6:226.

11. Cf. Beck, *A Commentary on Kant's "Critique of Practical Reason,"* pp. 176–81, 198–99, 202.

12. *M.P.R.*, p. 11; Ak. 6:213.

13. Ibid., p. 26; Ak. 6:226.

14. *F.M.M.*, p. 38n; Ak. 4:420n. Cf. *C.Pr.R.*, pp. 17–19; Ak. 5:18–21.

15. *M.P.R.*, p. 25; Ak. 6:225 (my emphasis). In the second *Critique*, Kant defines the will of rational beings as the "faculty of determining their causality through the conception of a rule" (*C.Pr.R.*, p. 32; Ak. 5:32). For the definition of a maxim, cf., in particular, *F.M.M.*, pp. 17n, 38n; Ak. 4:400n, 420n. "The [maxim] contains the practical rule *which reason determines* according to the conditions of the subject" (*F.M.M.*, p. 38; Ak. 4:420) (my emphasis).

16. "A maxim is a subjective principle of action which the subject adopts as a rule for himself (namely, how he wants to act). On the other hand, a principle of duty is that which reason absolutely and, therefore, objectively commands (how he should act)" (*M.P.R.*, pp. 25–26; Ak. 6:225). Cf. *C.Pr.R.*, p. 17; Ak. 5:19.

17. We shall see that when the object is nothing less than the moral law, the faculty of the human will is in reality a nonfaculty—an incapacity.

18. *C.Pr.R.*, p. 62; Ak. 5:60.

19. Ibid., p. 74; Ak. 5:72.

20. *Religion*, p. 19; Ak. 6:23–24.

21. *Education*, p. 83; Ak. 9:480.

22. *Opus Postumum*, Ak. 21:470: "We only know the freedom (of free choice) as a negative characteristic, as independence with respect to mo-

tives determining it according to pleasure or pain, in conformity or in opposition to the law (outside of the will). It always has the power, incomprehensible for us, to *resist* these motives (in themselves neither good nor bad) and *not merely the power to choose among them"* (my emphasis).

23. J. R. Silber, "The Ethical Significance of Kant's *Religion,"* Introductory Essay to Kant's *Religion,* trans. Theodore M. Greene and Hoyt H. Hudson (New York: Harper & Row, 1960), p. xcv: "The human *Willkür* is influenced but not wholly determined by impulses: its actions are always determined according to the strongest impulse, but only after the *Willkür* itself has made the decision by which the strongest impulse is determined."

24. *Religion,* p. 19; Ak. 6:24.
25. Cf. *C.Pr.R.,* p. 74; Ak. 5:72.
26. *M.P.R.,* p. 12; Ak. 6:213.
27. *C.P.R.,* p. 633; Ak. A802=B830 (my emphasis).
28. *M.P.R.,* p. 12; Ak. 6:213 (my emphasis).
29. Ibid.
30. *C.Pr.R.,* p. 30; Ak. 5:30.
31. Cf. *Religion,* p. 45 n; Ak. 6:49 n.

The concept of the freedom of the will [*Willkür*] does not precede the consciousness of the moral law in us. . . . Of this we can soon be convinced by asking ourselves whether we are certainly and immediately conscious of power to overcome, by a firm resolve, every incentive, *however great* [my emphasis], to transgression. . . . Everyone will have to admit that he *does not know* whether, were such a situation to arise, he would not be shaken in his resolution. Still, duty commands him absolutely: he *ought* to remain true to his resolve; and thence he rightly *concludes* [*schliesst*] that he must *be able* to do so, and that his will [*Willkür*] is therefore free.

32. *Religion,* p. 21 n; Ak. 6:26 n (my emphasis).
33. *C.Pr.R.,* pp. 99–100; Ak. 5:96 (my emphasis).
34. *M.P.R.,* p. 12; Ak. 6:213: "The will [*Wille*] is the faculty of desire regarded not (like choice [*Willkür*]) in relation to action, but rather as the ground determining choice to action."
35. *Religion,* p. 45 n; Ak. 6:49 n.
36. *M.P.R.,* p. 12; Ak. 6:213.
37. Ibid., p. 21; Ak. 6:221.
38. *Von einem neuerdings erhobenen vornehmen Ton in der philosophie,* Ak. 8:397 n.
39. *C.Pr.R.,* p. 36; Ak. 5:35. Cf. ibid., pp. 160–63; Ak. 5:156–59.
40. *C.F.J.,* p. 45; Ak. 5:210.
41. *Theory-Practice,* p. 49; Ak. 8:282. The expression "law of the freely choosing will" should not surprise the reader, since the law arises, not from the *Willkür,* but from the *Wille.* In fact Kant generally employs other expressions, such as "law of reason" or "law of the will [*Wille*]." Nevertheless, it is

not by accident that Kant in this case speaks plainly of the "law of the freely choosing will," since the context clearly indicates that Kant here treats the *maxim*, which can be good or bad according to whether the *Willkür* adopts the law as an incentive. The moral law *becomes* the law of free choice when the latter incorporates it into its maxim as an incentive. In light of the interest this expression holds for us, it seems useful to cite the passage in which it appears at length: "The maxim that a categorically commanding law of the freely choosing will should be observed absolutely, regardless of underlying ends (that is, duty) differs essentially, i.e., *in kind,* from the maxim to pursue an end supplied by nature itself as our motive for some sort of action (the end generally called happiness). For the first is good in itself, while the second is far from it; in the event of a clash with duty, it may be very evil."

42. *Anfang der Menschengeschichte,* Ak. 8:112 (my emphasis).

43. *F.M.M.,* p. 29; Ak. 4:412.

44. *C.Pr.R.,* p. 82; Ak. 5:72 (my emphasis).

45. Nabert, *L'Expérience intérieure,* pp. 307–9 (my emphasis).

46. *M.P.R.,* p. 27; Ak. 6:227.

47. Ibid., p. 12; Ak. 6:213.

48. Ibid.

49. Karl Leonhard Reinhold, *Briefe über die Kantische Philosophie* 2:272 (cited by Delbos, *La philosophie pratique de Kant,* p. 368 n. 2).

50. Reinhold's interpretation has the merit of reminding us that, according to Kant, the will is free even when it does evil. However, we must examine why this freedom to choose evil is in reality an incapacity of our freedom. Reinhold's error is in subordinating the freedom of the *Wille* to that of the *Willkür* and considering that the latter is more fundamental than the former.

51. *C.Pr.R.,* p. 32; Ak. 5:32.

52. *Opus Postumum,* Ak. 22:111–31.

53. *C.Pr.R.,* p. 33; Ak. 5:32. In this text, Kant employs the term *Willkür* when we would expect *Wille,* since it is a matter of the divine will. Cf. Delbos, *La philosophie pratique de Kant,* p. 351 n. Later in the second *Critique,* Kant will assert, "All three concepts—of incentive, interest, and maxim— . . . cannot, therefore, be applied to the divine will" (*C.Pr.R.,* p. 82; Ak. 5:141).

54. Cf. *F.M.M.,* p. 52; Ak. 4:434.

55. *Religion,* p. 45 n; Ak. 6:50 n.

56. *F.M.M.,* p. 29; Ak. 6:413.

57. The passage from the *Religion* previously cited establishes an equation between the contingency of action and indeterminism. Cf. *Religion,* p. 45 n; Ak. 6:50 n.

58. *F.M.M.,* p. 16; Ak. 4:400.

59. *Religion*, p. 20; Ak. 6:24.

60. *Versuch den Begriff der negativen Grössen in den Weltweisheit einzuführen,*
Ak. 2:177. Cf. *Religion*, p. 18 n; Ak. 6:22 n.

61. Ibid. Ak. 2:176–77.

62. *Religion*, p. 18 n; Ak. 6:23 n (added in the second addition). In *The
Metaphysical Principles of Right*, moreover, Kant writes: "An action which is
neither commanded nor prohibited is merely allowed, because for it there
is no law which limits freedom (authorization) and therefore also no duty.
Such an action is called morally indifferent (*indifferens, adiaphoron, res merae
facultatis*). It may be asked whether there are any such actions" (*M.P.R.*,
p. 23; Ak. 6:223).

63. *Opus Postumum*, Ak. 21:270.

64. *M.P.R.*, pp. 26–27; Ak. 6:226.

65. *Opus Postumum*, Ak. 21:470. We do not think there are grounds to
refer to the distinction between *Wille* and *Willkür* in the way Lewis White
Beck does: "The freedom of *Wille* is distinguished from that of *Willkür* as
libertas noumenon from *libertas phaenomenon*; yet the latter is not to be defined
empirically (cf. *Metaphysik der Sitten*, 6:226; and *Opus postumum*, 21:470), for
this gives only a comparative or psychological sense of freedom." He adds
that "Kant's statements are so cryptic that it is hard to know whether he is
entirely consistent or not" (Beck, *A Commentary on Kant's "Critique of Practical
Reason,"* p. 191 n. 43). On this point, see Rousset, *La doctrine kantienne de
l'objectivité*, p. 532 n. 2.

66. *C.Pr.R.*, p. 101; Ak. 5:97.

67. From the beginning of the first part of the *Religion*, Kant already
implies that man's choice is disposed to evil. While it is a question of the use
or abuse of free choice which makes man good or wicked by nature, Kant
does not hesitate to pursue this further by telling us that "the *source of evil*
[my emphasis] cannot lie . . . in a natural impulse; it can lie only in a rule
made by the will [*Willkür*]" (*Religion*, p. 17; Ak. 6:21). In section 2, he describes the propensity to evil before having established that man is wicked
by nature. Finally, certain passages from section 4 may apply to nontemporal choice in general, not merely to the choice of radical evil.

68. See *Religion*, p. 18; Ak. 6:22.

69. Ibid., p. 20; Ak. 6:25 (my emphasis).

70. Ibid., p. 21; Ak. 6:25.

71. Ibid., p. 17; Ak. 6:21.

72. Ibid., p. 26; Ak. 6:31.

73. Ibid., p. 17; Ak. 6:21.

74. Ibid., p. 17 n; Ak. 6:21 n.

75. Ibid., pp. 20, 17 n; Ak. 6:25, 21 n.

76. Ibid., pp. 39, 39 n; Ak. 6:21, 21 n.

77. Ibid., p. 17 n; Ak. 6 : 21 n.
78. Ibid., p. 21; Ak. 6 : 25.
79. Ibid.
80. Ibid., p. 17; Ak. 6 : 22.
81. Ibid., p. 24; Ak. 6 : 29.
82. Ibid., p. 20; Ak. 6 : 25. In this passage the term "inborn" is thus opposed, not to "acquired," but to "acquired in time."
83. Ibid., p. 17; Ak. 6 : 21.
84. Ibid., p. 20; Ak. 6 : 25 (my emphasis).
85. Ibid., p. 16; Ak. 6 : 20–21.
86. Ibid., p. 16; Ak. 6 : 21.
87. Ibid., p. 21; Ak. 6 : 25.
88. Cf. Ricoeur, *Conflict of Interpretations*, pp. 422, 434.
89. *Religion*, p. 25; Ak. 6 : 29.
90. Ibid., p. 26; Ak. 6 : 31.
91. Ibid., p. 32; Ak. 6 : 37.
92. Ibid., p. 30; Ak. 6 : 35.
93. Cf. *Anthropology*, p. 241; Ak. 7 : 324. Cf. Kant, *Réflexions sur l'éducation*, trans. A. Philonenko (Paris: Vrin, 1966), p. 34 n. 45.
94. *Religion*, p. 16; Ak. 6 : 21.
95. *Anthropology*, p. 203; Ak. 7 : 292.
96. *Religion*, p. 24; Ak. 6 : 28.
97. Ibid.
98. According to Weil, "the first two predispositions can be diverted from their end; only the third can divert them from it" (Weil, *Problèmes kantiens*, p. 156). This formulation is appealing, but it does not seem to us to reflect Kant's thought faithfully; indeed, did not Kant maintain that "it is absolutely impossible to graft anything evil" on the third predisposition (*Religion*, p. 23; Ak. 6 : 28)?
99. *Religion*, pp. 23, 40; Ak. 6 : 28, 44.
100. Ibid., p. 40; Ak. 6 : 44 (my emphasis).
101. Ibid., p. 40 n; Ak. 6 : 44 n.
102. Cf. Delbos, *La philosophie pratique de Kant*, p. 494: "Certainly the act of determining itself merely out of respect for the law cannot be regarded as the result of a natural predisposition, since it is meaningful only because of the freedom from which it proceeds; but it would no longer be possible if it were not related to a predisposition of this type."
103. *M.P.R.*, p. 23; Ak. 6 : 223. Cf. *C.Pr.R.*, p. 89; Ak. 5 : 86: "personality, i.e., . . . freedom."
104. *Religion*, pp. 27, 30; Ak. 6 : 32, 35.
105. Ibid., p. 26; Ak. 6 : 31.
106. Ibid.

107. Cf. n. 123 below on the difficulty which this position entails with respect to the affirmation of the reality of radical evil. On the problem of accountability, cf. Reboul, *Kant et le problème du mal*, pp. 148–62.

108. *Religion*, p. 16; Ak. 6:20. Cf. *C.P.R.*, pp. 475–79; Ak. A551–57=B579–85.

109. *C.Pr.R.*, p. 103; Ak. 5:100 (my emphasis).

110. Cf. *Religion*, p. 32; Ak. 6:37.

111. Jaspers, "Le mal radical chez Kant," p. 238.

112. *C.Pr.R.*, p. 103; Ak. 5:99.

113. Arthur Schopenhauer, *On the Basis of Morality*, trans. E. F. J. Payne (Indianapolis: Bobbs-Merrill Company, 1965), p. 112.

114. *C.Pr.R.*, p. 101; Ak. 5:98 (my emphasis).

115. Plato, *Republic*, 10:614a.

116. *C.Pr.R.*, p. 98; Ak. 5:94 (my emphasis).

117. Ibid.

118. Schopenhauer, *On the Basis of Morality*, p. 112.

119. *C.Pr.R.*, p. 38; Ak. 5:36 (my emphasis).

120. *C.P.R.*, p. 477; Ak. A555=B583 (my emphasis).

121. *Religion*, p. 45 n; Ak. 6:50 n (my emphasis).

122. Ibid., p. 36; Ak. 6:41.

123. *Religion*, p. 28; Ak. 6:32–33. Delbos underscores what would seem to be a surprising contradiction in Kant's thought. In effect, Kant argues that we can never decide, on the basis of the experience of actions contrary to the law, that the one who did them is himself wicked. Cf. Delbos, *La philosophie pratique de Kant*, p. 498.

124. Ibid., p. 35; Ak. 6:40.

125. Ibid., p. 27; Ak. 6:32 (my emphasis).

126. Ibid. Cf. ibid., pp. 16, 20, 24; Ak. 6:21, 25, 29. The universality of this evil [*die Allgemeinheit dieses Bösen*] (*Religion*, pp. 25, 27; Ak. 6:30, 32) is a universality of the act, for evil is contingent in man. The expression "man is evil by nature" (*Religion*, p. 27; Ak. 6:32) means that *all men freely* contract the propensity to evil and that this propensity, while subjectively necessary in every man, must nevertheless be imputed to each.

127. Ibid., pp. 24, 32; Ak. 6:29, 37.

128. Ibid., p. 38; Ak. 6:43 (my emphasis).

129. Ibid., p. 32; Ak. 6:37.

130. Ibid., p. 26; Ak. 6:31.

131. Ibid.

132. *Anfang der Menschengeschichte*, Ak. 8:123 (my emphasis).

133. *Religion*, pp. 35–36; Ak. 6:40–41 (my emphasis). Cf. Ricoeur, *Conflict of Interpretations*, p. 435:

Evil would cease to be evil if it ceased to be "a manner of being of freedom, which itself comes from freedom." Therefore, evil does not have an origin in the sense of an antecedent cause. "In the search for the rational origin of evil actions, every such action must be regarded as though the individual had fallen into it directly from a state of innocence." Everything is in this "as if." It is the philosophical equivalent of the myth of the Fall; it is the rational myth of the coming-to-be of evil, of the instantaneous passage from innocence to sin; *as* Adam—rather than *in* Adam—we originate evil.

134. *Anfang der Menschengeschichte,* Ak. 8 : 123 (my emphasis).

135. *Religion,* p. 17; Ak. 6 : 21.

136. Nabert, *L'experiénce intérieure,* pp. 211 – 12. Cf. Karl Barth, *Church Dogmatics,* vol. 4, pt. 1, trans. G. W. Bromiley (Edinburgh: T & T Clark, 1956), 495:

In relation to the transgression and therefore the corruption of man there is no time in which man is not a transgressor and therefore guiltless before God. To use the phrase of Kant, he lives by an "evil principle," with a "bias towards evil," in the power of a "radical evil" which shows itself virulent and active in his life, with which in some incomprehensible but actual way he accepts solidarity, with which he is not identical, but to which he commits himself and is committed. He transgresses because he continually derives from the transgression which—against his nature, in a way which is foreign to himself, in flagrant contradiction with himself—he commits in and with the fact that he is. The very fact that he is means that he transgresses: *against himself, but by and of himself, denying and forfeiting his freedom,* which is a freedom for God and his neighbour and no other; but as his own act and being, the way to captivity which he himself has gone" (my emphasis).

137. *Opus Postumum,* Ak. 21 : 471. Cf. *M.P.R.,* p. 26; Ak. 6 : 226.

138. Cf. *C.Pr.R.,* p. 31; Ak. 5 : 31.

139. Cf. *Religion,* p. 26; Ak. 6 : 31.

140. *M.P.R.,* Ak. 6 : 321 n.

141. *Religion,* p. 26; Ak. 6 : 31.

142. Ibid., p. 34 n; Ak. 6 : 39 n.

143. Ibid., p. 27, Ak: 6 : 32.

144. Ibid., p. 38; Ak. 6 : 43.

145. *Opus Postumum,* Ak. 21 : 470.

146. *M.P.R.,* p. 26, Ak: 6 : 226.

147. *Religion,* p. 38; Ak. 6 : 43.

148. Ibid., p. 32; Ak. 6 : 37.

149. Ibid., p. 38; Ak. 6 : 43. Cf. Paul Ricoeur, *History and Truth,* trans. Charles A. Kelbley (Evanston, Ill.: Northwestern University Press, 1965), p. 300.

150. *Religion,* p. 25; Ak. 6 : 30.

151. Ibid., p. 24; Ak. 6 : 29.

152. On this subject, cf. Bruch's interesting interpretation, Bruch, *La philosophie religieuse de Kant,* pp. 67 – 68. We still question whether there are not grounds to seek to *justify* the place to which Kant assigns this passage

158   *Notes to Pages 105–108*

within the first chapter of the *Religion,* rather than speak, as Bruch does, of "the *artificiality* of the enterprise of describing the propensity to evil before having established the origin and reality of evil" (p. 68).

153. Rom. 7:19.

154. *Theory-Practice,* p. 49; Ak. 8:282.

155. *F.M.M.,* p. 77; Ak. 4:457–58. Cf. *Religion,* pp. 29–30; Ak. 6:34–35. Cf. *Preisschrift über die Fortschritte der Metaphysik,* Ak. 20:346 (loose sheets). Cf. *M.P.R.,* Ak. 6:321 n: "Every violation of the law can and must be explained only as deriving from a maxim adopted by the wrongdoer (that of taking the action as a rule), for if it derived from some sensible propensity, he would not be the author of it as a *free* being, and it could not be imputed to him."

156. *Religion,* p. 30; Ak. 6:35. Cf. *F.M.M.,* p. 65; Ak. 4:446: "The concept of a causality entails that of laws."

157. *Religion,* p. 32; Ak. 6:37.

158. *C.Pr.R.,* p. 32; Ak. 5:32 (my emphasis).

159. *Religion,* p. 31; Ak. 6:36.

160. This is why we do not think we are obliged to subscribe to the formula of Gilles Deleuze, which has it that, according to Kant, "when we choose against the law . . . [w]e cease to be subjects, but primarily because we cease to be legislators (indeed we take the law which determines us from sensibility)" (G. Deleuze, *Kant's Critical Philosophy,* trans. Hugh Tomlinson and Barbara Habberjam [Minneapolis: University of Minnesota Press, 1984], pp. 32–33). It is important to distinguish between the law that the will promulgates as having a universal value (the moral law) and the law by which the will is determined (which could either be the moral law or a pathological law, according to which the will realizes or fails to realize its autonomy). When there is a heteronomy of free choice, "the will does not give itself the law but only directions for a reasonable obedience to pathological laws" (*C.Pr.R.,* p. 34; Ak. 5:59); in doing so the will does not cease being legislative, yet even while recognizing the validity of the categorical imperative, it permits itself to deviate from it. "When we observe ourselves in any transgression of a duty, we find that we do not actually will that our maxim should become a universal law. That is impossible for us; rather, the contrary of this maxim should remain as a law generally" (*F.M.M.,* p. 42; Ak. 4:424).

161. *F.M.M.,* p. 74; Ak. 4:455.

162. *M.P.V.,* p. 37 n; Ak. 6:380 nn.

163. *C.Pr.R.,* p. 64; Ak. 5:62. Cf. *F.M.M.,* pp. 55, 58; Ak. 4:437, 439.

164. *Religion,* p. 30; Ak. 6:35.

165. This was already indicated by the description of the propensity to evil when we considered the first degree of that propensity—the frailty of human nature. Cf. *Religion,* p. 25; Ak. 6:29.

166. Cf. *Religion,* p. 25; Ak. 6:30 for the description of the third degree of the propensity to evil—the wickedness of the human heart.

167. Cf. *Religion,* p. 25; Ak. 6:30 for the description of the second degree of the propensity to evil—the impurity of the human heart.

168. *Religion,* p. 32; Ak. 6:26. Cf. ibid., p. 45; Ak. 6:50.

169. Ibid., p. 37; Ak. 6:42.

170. Nabert, *Essai sur le mal,* pp. 77–78.

Chapter Six

1. *Religion,* p. 32; Ak. 6:37.

2. Ibid., p. 39; Ak. 6:44.

3. *C.Pr.R.,* p. 40; Ak. 5:38 (my emphasis).

4. *Religion,* p. 41; Ak. 6:45. The expression "seed of goodness" appears several times in Kant's writings. The opinion of those moralists who maintain that the world progresses from evil toward good appears to him to be a "well-intentioned assumption" intended to "encourage the sedulous cultivation of that seed of goodness which perhaps lies in us" (*Religion,* p. 16; Ak. 6:20). In another passage, Kant asserts that radical evil "constitutes the foul taint in our race. So long as we do not eradicate [*herausbringen*] it, it prevents the seed of goodness from developing as it otherwise would" (*Religion,* p. 34; Ak. 6:38).

5. Jaspers, "Le mal radical chez Kant," p. 241.

6. *Religion,* p. 32; Ak. 6:37.

7. Ibid. Cf. ibid., p. 26; Ak. 6:31. If it is impossible to extirpate [*vertilgen* (Ak. 6:37), *ausrotten* (Ak. 6:31)] radical evil by human power, it must nevertheless be possible to overcome it [*überwiegen* (Ak. 6:37)].

8. Ibid., p. 35; Ak. 6:40.

9. Ibid., pp. 45–46; Ak. 6:50.

10. Ibid., p. 46; Ak. 6:51 (my emphasis).

11. Ibid.

12. Ibid., p. 40; Ak. 6:44.

13. Nabert, *Essai sur le mal,* p. 164.

14. *Religion,* p. 39; Ak. 6:44 (my emphasis).

15. Ibid., p. 46; Ak. 6:51.

16. *Confl. Fac.,* p. 107; Ak. 7:59.

17. Ibid., pp. 75–77; Ak. 7:43–44 (my emphasis).

18. *Religion,* p. 47; Ak. 6:52 (my emphasis). Cf. *Confl. Fac.,* p. 77; Ak. 7:44.

19. *Religion,* p. 41; Ak. 6:45. Cf. the outline of a letter intended for Lavater (ca. 1775) where Kant says,

What is essential and excellent in Christ's doctrine is precisely that he placed the sum of religion in the act of integrating all one's strength in one's faith, that is, in the unconditional confidence that God will, in what follows, complete that part of the good which is not in our power. This doctrine forbids any claim to know how God will accomplish it; in the same way it forbids the presumptuous temerity of deciding what means are most comfortable to his wisdom, and similarly every attempt to seek his favor according to the established rules of the religious cult. Nothing remains of the infinite religious illusion, to which men are at all times inclined in the matter of religion, than the general and indeterminate confidence that this good will be imparted to us in some manner, and to the extent that we do not by our conduct render ourselves unworthy (Ak. 10:179–80. Cited by Weil, *Problèmes kantiens*, p. 145).

20. *Religion*, p. 47; Ak. 6:52. Cf. *Confl. Fac.*, p. 77; Ak. 7:44.
21. Ibid.
22. *Confl. Fac.*, p. 75; Ak. 7:43.
23. *Religion*, p. 46; Ak. 6:51.
24. Ibid., p. 47; Ak. 6:52.
25. Ibid., p. 40; Ak. 6:44.
26. *Opus Postumum*, Ak. 21:34. Cf. ibid., 66.
27. *Religion*, p. 40; Ak. 6:45.
28. *M.P.V.*, p. 56; Ak. 6:397.
29. *C.Pr.R.*, p. 137; Ak. 5:132.
30. Cf. Ricoeur's interpretation in *The Conflict of Interpretations*, p. 422:

What the *Essay on Radical Evil* teaches about freedom, indeed, is that this same power that duty imputes to us is in reality a nonpower; . . . The nonpower signified by radical evil is discovered in the very place whence our power proceeds. Thus is posed in radical terms the question of the real causality of our freedom, the very same freedom which the *Practical Reason* postulated at the end of its Dialectic. The "postulate" of freedom must henceforth cross through, not only the night of knowing, with its crisis of the transcendental illusion, but also the night of power, with its crisis of radical evil.

31. Kant to Lavater, 28 April 1775, Ak. 10:176.
32. The "Essay on Radical Evil" of 1793 could well have surprised, even scandalized Kant's contemporaries, but for Kant himself it contained nothing new. Cf., on this subject, Weil, *Problème kantiens*, pp. 143 ff.
33. *C.Pr.R.*, p. 111; Ak. 5:106–7.
34. Ibid., p. 115; Ak. 5:110.
35. Ricoeur, *Conflict of Interpretations*, p. 417.
36. *C.Pr.R.*, p. 138; Ak. 5:133.
37. Ibid., p. 113; Ak. 5:109.
38. Ibid.
39. Ibid., p. 134; Ak. 5:129. Cf. ibid., pp. 117–24; Ak. 5:113–19.
40. Ibid., p. 118; Ak. 5:114.
41. *C.F.J.*, p. 323 n; Ak. 5:471 n.
42. *C.Pr.R.*, p. 118; Ak. 5:114.
43. Ibid., p. 149 n; Ak. 5:143 n. Cf. ibid., p. 148; Ak. 5:143: "The subjective effect of this law, i.e., the intention which is suitable to this law and

which is necessary because of it, the intention to promote the practically possible highest good at least presupposes that the latter is possible. Otherwise it would be practically impossible to strive for the object of a concept, which, at bottom, would be empty and without an object." Cf. also *C.Pr.R.*, p. 150; Ak. 5:144: "Now with respect to the first component of the highest good, viz. morality, the moral law merely gives a command, and to doubt the possibility of that ingredient would be the same as to call the moral law itself into question."

44. Ibid., pp. 116, 120; Ak. 5:112, 116.

45. Ibid., p. 148; Ak. 5:142.

46. For a study of the relations between the three postulates, cf. Ricoeur, "Freedom in the Light of Hope," in *Conflict of Interpretations*, pp. 402–24.

47. *C.Pr.R.*, p. 127; Ak. 5:122 (my emphasis).

48. Ibid., p. 137; Ak. 5:132.

49. *Logic*, p. 119; Ak. 9:112.

50. Ibid., p. 149n; Ak. 5:143n.

51. Ibid., p. 12n; Ak. 5:11n.

52. *Logic*, p. 119; Ak. 9:112.

53. *C.F.J.*, p. 324n; Ak. 5:471n.

54. Ibid., p. 301n; Ak. 5:450n.

55. Ibid., p. 325; Ak. 5:472.

56. *C.Pr.R.*, p. 130; Ak. 5:125.

57. Ibid.

58. Rousset, in *La doctrine kantienne*, pp. 545–53, clearly sets out the "*logical need* for coherence" (p. 546n) in reason, which forces it to grant the conditions necessary to the reality of its practical object; it seems to me, however, that there is no reason to state this aspect of Kant's thought so strongly, and to trace everything—or nearly everything—back to a logical requirement. Thus when Kant speaks of the "interest of reason" (cf. *C.Pr.R.*, p. 125; Ak. 5:120) it seems to me that the phrase "logical interest" of reason (Rousset, *La doctrine kantienne*, p. 549) must be taken to mean "the interest of reason in its own rationality" (Rousset, *La doctrine kantienne*, p. 546). It is a matter of the *practical* interest of reason which impels it, not to assure its own coherence, but to *make objects actual* (cf. *C.P.R.*, p. 18; Ak. 3:x). "Every interest is ultimately practical," Kant says (*C.Pr.R.*, p. 126; Ak. 5:121), which indicates that in the end reason's interest is not in knowing but in acting. Cf. Deleuze, *Kant's Critical Philosophy*, pp. 5–7, 25–27, et passim. Cf. Burgelin, "Kant et les fins de la raison," p. 145.

59. *C.F.J.*, p. 324n; Ak. 5:471n.

61. *C.Pr.R.*, pp. 130, 149–50; Ak. 5:126, 5:144; "What is Orientation in Thinking?" pp. 299–300; Ak. 8:140–41.

62. Ibid., p. 152; Ak. 5:147.

63. *C.F.J.*, p. 324; Ak. 5:471.

64. *C.Pr.R.*, p. 148; Ak. 5:142.

65. "What is Orientation in Thinking?" p. 298; Ak. 8:139.

66. Cf. ibid.

67. *C.Pr.R.*, p. 148; Ak. 5:143. On the distinction between a hypothesis and a postulate, cf. "What is Orientation in Thinking?" pp. 299–302; Ak. 8:140–42; *C.Pr.R.*, pp. 145–49; Ak. 5:140–44; and A. Philonenko's introduction to his French translation of "What is Orientation in Thinking?" pp. 67–68.

68. Cf. *C.Pr.R.*, p. 148; Ak. 5:143.

69. Ibid., p. 130; Ak. 5:125.

70. Ibid., p. 149; Ak. 5:144.

71. Ibid., p. 130; Ak. 5:125.

72. Ibid., p. 12 n; Ak. 5:11 n.

73. Ibid.

74. *C.P.R.*, p. 650; Ak. 4:829 or 3:857.

75. Ibid.

76. Ibid.

77. Cf. *C.Pr.R.*, p. 159; Ak. 5:143: "The righteous man may say: I will that there be a God." It is a free step, "about which we have a choice" (*C.Pr.R.*, p. 150; Ak. 5:145). "The manner in which we are to think of it as possible is subject to our own choice" (*C.Pr.R.*, p. 151; Ak. 5:145). "The principle which here determines our judgment . . . is a faith of pure practical reason . . . a voluntary decision of our judgment" (*C.Pr.R.*, p. 151; Ak. 5:146). This is why when he speaks of the "promise of the moral law," Kant specifies that it does not concern a promise "*contained* in it," but a promise "such as I *put* into it [*hineinlege*] and that on morally adequate grounds" (*C.F.J.*, p. 324n; Ak. 5:462 n. 2) (my emphasis). Cf. on this point, Rousset, *La doctrine kantienne*, pp. 549–50.

78. Cf. n. 84 below.

79. Cf. *C.Pr.R.*, p. 49; Ak. 5:48.

80. Cf. ibid., p. 140; Ak. 5:135.

81. Ibid., p. 4; Ak. 5:4.

82. See *C.Pr.R.*, p. 143; Ak. 5:138. Cf. *C.Pr.R.*, p. 151; Ak. 5:145–46.

83. Ibid., p. 130; Ak. 5:126.

84. Cf. *C.F.J.*, p. 321; Ak. 5:469: "This commanded effect, *together with the only* [*den einzigen*] *conditions of its possibility thinkable by us*, viz. the Being of God and the immortality of the soul, are *things of faith* (*res fidei*) and of all objects are the only ones [*die einzigen*] which can be so called." This is not the only passage where Kant does not include freedom among the postulates. In particular, cf. *C.Pr.R.*, p. 12 n; Ak. 5:11 n.

85. Cf. *C.Pr.R.*, p. 50; Ak. 5:49 (my emphasis).

86. *C.P.R.*, p. 650; Ak. 4:829 or 3:857.

87. Delbos, *La philosophie pratique de Kant*, p. 400. L. Brunschvicg also adopts Delbos's thesis (cf. Brunschvicg, *Écrits philosophiques*, 1:198, 1:253–54). Gueroult, on the other hand, opposes it (cf. Gueroult, "L'antidogmatisme de Kant et de Fichte," pp. 222–24). For Gueroult, "the affirmation of the existence of Freedom in the name of the moral law is contained strictly in the definition of a postulate" (p. 223). We cannot agree with this. The postulated ideas are the object of a lesser certitude than that accorded to the moral law, and hence to freedom as identical to the moral law. In support of Delbos's positions, cf. Alquié, *La morale de Kant*, pp. 99–101, and Ricoeur, *Conflict of Interpretations*, pp. 418–19.

88. *C.Pr.R.*, p. 122; Ak. 5:117. Cf. *C.Pr.R.*, p. 137; Ak. 5:132. Kant, we said (p. 118 above), places the freedom which is postulated at the same level as the ideas of God and immortality. It now seems that we must qualify this claim, for there the place and role assigned to freedom seemed unique. At first glance, we were tempted to think that Kant accorded greater importance to the postulates of God and immortality, since he never fails to name them, whether he names only these two (as he does repeatedly), or adds a third (which is not always that of freedom). (Cf. Delbos, *La philosophie pratique de Kant*, pp. 397–98.) Moreover, the postulates of God and immortality cannot have any meaning if we also grant that there is in us, despite our fall into radical evil, "a capacity for following the moral law with an unyielding disposition." Hence it is with justice, but not without paradox, that Ricoeur maintains that "[postulated] freedom is the true pivot of the doctrine of the postulates. . . . The other two postulates . . . serve only to make explicit the potential of hope of the postulate of existential freedom" (Ricoeur, *Conflict of Interpretations*, pp. 419–20).

89. *Progress*, p. 123; Ak. 20:295.

90. *Verkündigung des nahen Abschlusses eines Tractats zum ewigen Frieden in der Philosophie*, Ak. 8:418.

91. *M.P.V.*, pp. 40–41; Ak. 6:383.

92. Delbos, *Bulletin de la Société francaise de philosophie*, p. 15.

93. *Progress*, p. 125; Ak. 20:295.

94. *Religion*, p. 25; Ak. 6:31.

95. *M.P.V.*, p. 37; Ak. 6:380 (my emphasis).

96. Delbos, in *Bulletin de la Société francaise de philosophie*, p. 15.

97. *Religion*, p. 32; Ak. 6:37. Cf. *Religion*, p. 26; Ak. 6:31.

98. *M.P.R.*, p. 41; Ak. 6:383.

99. *C.Pr.R.*, p. 87; Ak. 5:84.

100. Ibid., pp. 4, 150; Ak. 5:7, 5:260.

Bibliography

Alexandre, M. *Lecture de Kant.* Texts collected and annotated by G. Granel. Paris: Presses Universitaires de France, 1961.

Alquié, F. *La morale de Kant.* Paris: Centre de documentation universitaire, 1959.

—. *La critique kantienne de la métaphysique.* Paris: Presses Universitaires de France, 1968.

Barth, Karl. *Church Dogmatics.* Vol. 4, pt. 1. Translated by G. W. Bromiley. Edinburgh: T & T Clark, 1956.

Barthélemy-Madaule, M. *Bergson adversaire de Kant.* Paris: Presses Universitaires de France, 1966.

Baumgarten, A. G. *Megaphysica.* 7th ed. Reprint. Hidesheim: Georg Olms, 1963.

Beck, L. W. "Apodictic Imperatives." *Kantstudien* 49 (1957): 7–24.

—. "Les deux concepts kantiens du vouloir dan leur contexte politique." *Annales de philosophie politique* 4 (1962): 119–37.

—. *Studies in the Philosophy of Kant.* New York: Liberal Arts Press, 1965.

—. *A Commentary on Kant's "Critique of Practical Reason."* Chicago: University of Chicago Press, Phoenix Books, 1966.

Besse, G. *La morale selon Kant et selon Marx.* Paris: Centre d'études et de recherches marxistes, 1963.

Bohatec, J. *Die Religionsphilosophie Kants in der "Religion innerhalb der Grenzen der blossen Vernunft" mit besonderer Berücksichtigung ihrer theologisch-dogmatischen Quellen.* Hamburg: Hoffman und Campe, 1938.

Boutroux, E. *La philosophie de Kant.* Paris: Vrin, 1926.

Bruch, J.-L. *La philosophie religieuse de Kant.* Paris: Aubier, 1968.

Brunschvicg, L. *Écrits philosophiques.* Vol. 1, *L'humanisme de l'occident. Descartes, Spinoza, Kant.* Paris: Presses Universitaires de France, 1951.

—. *Le progrès de la conscience dans la philosophie occidentale.* 2 vols. Paris: Presses Universitaires de France, 1953.

Burgelin, P. "Kant et les fins de la raison." *Revue de métaphysique et de morale* 58 (Paris) (1953): 130–52.

Caird, E. *The Critical Philosophy of Immanuel Kant.* 2 vols. Glasgow: James Maclehose and sons, 1889. Reprint. New York: Kraus Reprint Co., 1968.

Cantecor, G. *Kant.* Paris: Éditions Mellotée, 1909.

Cassirer, H. W., *Kant's First Critique*. London: Georges Allen and Unwin; New York: Humanities Press, 1954.

Daudin, H. *La liberté de la volonté*. Paris: Presses Universitaires de France, 1950.

Daval, R. *La métaphysique de Kant*. Paris: Presses Universitaires de France, 1951.

Delbos, V. "Sur la formation de l'idée de jugement synthétique a priori chez Kant." *Année philosophique* (Paris) (1910): 13–34.

———. "Kant." Chapter 6 in *Figures et doctrines de philosophes*, 196–259. Paris: Plon, 1921.

———. *La philosophie pratique de Kant*. 3d ed. Paris: Presses Universitaires de France, 1969.

Deleuze, G. *Différence et répétition*. Paris: Presses Universitaires de France, 1968.

———. *Kant's Critical Philosophy*. Translated by Hugh Tomlinson and Barbara Habberjam. Minneapolis: University of Minnesota Press, 1984.

Duncan, A. R. C. *Practical Reason and Morality: A Study of Immanuel Kant's "Foundations for the Metaphysics of Morals."* London: Nelson, 1957.

Evellin, F. *La raison pure et les antinomies*. Paris: Alcan, 1907.

Goldmann, L. *La communauté humaine et l'univers chez Kant*. Paris: Presses Universitaires de France, 1948. Reprint. *Introduction à la philosophie de Kant*. Paris: Gallimard, 1967.

Granel, G. *L'équivoque ontologique de la pensée kantienne*. Paris: Gallimard, 1970.

———. "L'antidogmatisme de Kant et de Fichte." *Revue de métaphysique et de morale* 27 (Paris) (1920): 181–224.

———. *L'évolution et la structure de la doctrine de la science chez Fichte*. 2 vols. Paris: Les Belles Lettres, 1930.

———. "Canon de la raison pure et critique de la raison pratique." *Revue internationale de philosophie* (Brussels) 4 (1954): 331–57.

———. *Annuaire du Collège de France*. 1958–59 and 1959–60.

———. "Nature humaine et état de nature chez Rousseau, Kant et Fichte." *Les cahiers pour l'analyse* (Paris), no. 6 (1967): 1–19.

Guillermit, L. "Commentaire des Paralogismes." *Cahiers de philosophie de la faculté des lettres et sciences humaines de Paris*. Paris, 1963.

Guillermit, L., and J. Vuillemin. *Le Sens du destin*. Neuchâtel: Éditions de la Baconnière, 1948.

Havet, J. *Kant et la problème du temps*. Paris: Gallimard, 1946.

Heidegger, M. *Kant and the Problem of Metaphysics*. Translated by James S. Churchill. Bloomington: Indiana University Press, 1962.

Hoernle, A. "Kant's Theory of Freedom." *The Personalist* 20 (1939): 391–99.

Jaspers, K. "Le mal radical chez Kant." *Deucalion* 4, no. 36 (1952): 227–52.

————. *Les grands philosophes: Ceux qui fondent la philosophie et ne cessent de l'engendrer: Kant.* Translated by J. Hersch. Paris: Plon, 1967.

Julia, D. *La question de l'homme et le fondement de la philosophie.* Paris: Aubier, 1964.

Klein, Z. *La notion de dignité humaine dans la pensée de Kant et de Pascal.* Paris: Vrin, 1968.

Körner, S. *Kant.* Baltimore: Penguin Books, 1955.

————. "Kant's Conception of Freedom. Dawes Hicks Lecture on Philosophy." In *Proceedings of the British Academy,* vol. 53, pp. 193–217. London: Oxford University Press, 1967.

Krüger, G. *Critique et morale chez Kant.* Translated by M. Régnier. Paris: Beauchesne, 1961.

Lachelier, J. *Oeuvres de Jules Lachelier.* 2 vols. Paris: Alcan, 1933.

Lachièze-Rey, P. *L'idéalisme kantien.* 2d ed. Paris: Vrin, 1950.

Lacroix, J. "La philosophie kantienne de l'histoire." Chap. 2 in *Histoire et mystère: Cahiers de l'actualité religieuse.* Vol. 18. Paris: Casterman, 1962.

————. *Kant et le Kantisme.* Paris: Presses Universitaires de France, 1966.

Maréchal, J. *Le point de départ de la métaphysique.* Vol. 3, *La critique de Kant.* 4th ed. Brussels and Paris: Desclée de Brouwer, 1964.

————. *Le point de départ de la métaphysique.* Vol. 4, *Le système idéaliste chez Kant et les post-kantiens.* Brussels and Paris: Desclée de Brouwer, 1947.

Martin, G. *Science moderne et ontologie traditionnelle chez Kant.* Translated by J.-C. Piguet. Paris: Presses Universitaires de France, 1963.

Marty, F. "La typique du jugement pratique pur." *Archives de philosophie* 19 (October, 1955), pp. 56–87.

Moreau, J. "Kant et la morale." *Archives de philosophie* 25 (1962): 163–84.

————. *Le dieu des philosophes.* Paris: Vrin, 1969.

Mosse-Bastide, R.-M. *La liberté.* Paris: Presses Universitaires de France, 1966.

Muralt, A. de. *La conscience transcendantale dans le criticisme kantien.* Paris: Aubier, 1958.

Nabert, J. *L'expérience intérieure de la liberté.* Paris: Presses Universitaires de France, 1924.

————. "L'expérience interne chez Kant." *Revue de métaphysique et de morale* 31 (1924): 205–68.

————. *Essai sur le Mal.* Paris: Presses Universitaires de France, 1955.

Naulin, P. *L'itinéraire de la conscience.* Paris: Aubier, 1963.

Pascal, G. *Pour connaître la pensée de Kant.* Paris: Bordas, 1966.

Paton, H. J. *In Defense of Reason.* London: Hutchinson, 1951.

————. *Kant's Metaphysic of Experience.* 4th ed. 2 vols. London: George Allen and Unwin, 1965.

————. *The Categorical Imperative.* 6th ed. London: Hutchinson, 1967.

Philonenko, A. *La liberté humaine dans la philosophie de Fichte.* Paris: Vrin, 1966.

————. *Théorie et praxis dans la pensée morale et politique de Kant et de Fichte en 1793.* Paris: Vrin, 1968.

————. *L'oeuvre de Kant: La philosophie critique.* Vol. 1, *La philosophie précritique et la "Critique de la raison pure."* Paris: Vrin, 1969.

Reboul, O. "Prescription ou proscription? Essai sur le sens du devoir chez Kant." *Revue de métaphysique et de morale* 72 (1967): 295–320.

————. *Kant et le problème du mal.* Montréal: Presses de l'Université de Montréal, 1971.

Ricoeur, P. "Sympathie et respect: phénoménologie et éthique de la deuxième personne." *Revue de métaphysique et de morale* 59 (October–December 1954): 380–97.

————. *Fallible Man.* Translated by Charles A. Kelbley. Chicago: Henry Regnery, 1965.

————. *History and Truth.* Translated by Charles A. Kelbley. Evanston, Ill.: Northwestern University Press, 1965.

————. *Freedom and Nature: The Voluntary and the Involuntary.* Translated by Erazim V. Kohák. Evanston, Ill.: Northwestern University Press, 1966.

————. *The Symbolism of Evil.* Translated by Emerson Buchanon. New York: Harper and Row, 1967.

————. *The Conflict of Interpretations.* Edited by Don Ihde. Evanston, Ill.: Northwestern University Press, 1974.

Ross, D. *Kant's Ethical Theory: A Commentary on the "Grundlegung zur Metaphysik der Sitten."* Oxford: Clarendon Press, 1954.

Rousset, B. *La doctrine kantienne de l'objectivité.* Paris: Vrin, 1967.

Schaerer, R. "'Si dieu n'existe pas . . . ,' Réflexions sur Kant et Dostoïevsky." *Revue de théologie et de philosophie* 100 (1967): 93–110.

Schilpp, P. A. *Kant's Pre-critical Ethics.* 2d ed. Evanston, Ill.: Northwestern University Press, 1960.

Schopenhauer, A. *On the Basis of Morality.* Translated by E. F. J. Payne. Indianapolis: The Bobbs-Merrill Company, 1965.

————. *The World as Will and Representation.* Translated by E. F. J. Payne. New York: Dover Publications, 1969.

Sidgwick, H. "The Kantian Conception of Free Will." *Mind* 13 (1888): 405–12.

Silber, J. R. "The Ethical Significance of Kant's Religion." Introductory Essay to Kant's *Religion within the Limits of Reason Alone,* translated by Theodore M. Greene and Hoyt H. Hudson. New York: Harper & Row, 1960.

Smith, Norman Kemp. *A Commentary to Kant's "Critique of Pure Reason."* New York: Humanities Press, 1962.

Strawson, P. F. *The Bounds of Sense: An Essay on Kant's "Critique of Pure Reason."* London: Methuen and Co., 1966.

Ulmann, J. *La nature et l'éducation: L'idée de nature dans l'éducation physique et dans l'éducation morale.* Paris: Vrin, 1964.

Vaihinger, H. *The Philosophy of "As If."* Translated by C. K. Ogden. New York: Harcourt, Brace & Company, 1925.

Vancourt, R. *Kant.* Paris: Presses Universitaires de France, 1967.

Verneaux, R. *Le vocabulaire de Kant: Doctrines et méthodes.* Paris: Aubier, 1967.

Vialatoux, J. *La morale de Kant.* Paris: Presses Universitaires de France, 1956.

Vlachos, G. *La pensée politique de Kant.* Paris: Presses Universitaires de France, 1962.

Vleeschauwer, J.-J. de. "Les antinomies kantiennes et la Clavis universalis d'Arthur Collier." *Mind* n.s. 47 (1938): 303–20.

———. *L'évolution de la pensée kantienne.* Paris: Alcan, 1939.

———. "La doctrine du suicide dans l'éthique de Kant." *Kantstudien* 57 (1966): 251–66.

Vuillemin, J. *L'héritage kantien et la révolution copernicienne.* Paris: Presses Universitaires de France, 1954.

———. *Physique et métaphysique kantiennes.* Paris: Presses Universitaires de France, 1955.

Weil, E. *Problèmes kantiens.* 2d ed. Paris: Vrin, 1970.

Williams, T. C. *The Concept of the Categorical Imperative.* London: Clarendon Press, 1968.

Wolff, E. "Les trois impératifs catégoriques et les trois posulats de la raison pratique chez kant." *Archives de philosophie* 29 (1966): 37–58.

Zac, S. "Intention et action dans 'La religion dans les limites de la simple raison' de Kant." *Revue le l'enseignement philosophique* (February–March 1966): 1–8.

Index

Abbot, T. K., 151n. 6
Adiaphoron morale, 92
Aliquié, Ferdinand, 128n. 15, 138n. 38, 150n. 2
Als ob ["as if"], 23, 147n. 194
Analogy, second, 127n. 6 to chap. 1
Antinomies, 16, 23; dynamical and mathematical, 139n. 8 to chap. 3
Antinomy, 138n. 38; "lived," 14; fourth, 7; third, 3, 4, 6–8, 11–12, 15, 19, 36, 95, 143n. 102
Appearances, 4–6, 10–12, 23, 41, 53, 129n. 26, 136n. 22; ground of, 9; intelligible cause of, 9
Apperception, 34; nonempirical, 12
Autocracy, 119–20
Autonomy, 50, 51, 77; as a given and a task, 79

Barth, Karl, 157n. 136
Beck, Lewis White, 131n. 69, 132n. 93, 136n. 14, 138n. 24, 154n. 65
Bruch, Jean-Louis, 137n. 12, 157n. 152
Brunschvicg, Léon, 6

C.F.J. See *Kant's Critique of Judgment*
C.P.R. See *Immanuel Kant's Critique of Pure Reason*
C.Pr.R. See *Critique of Practical Reason*
Canon of Pure Reason, 16, 25, 131n. 70, 136n. 14, 140n. 23
Categorical imperative, 25, 46, 47, 49, 50, 51, 53, 54, 71, 79, 82, 89, 114, 140nn. 23, 29, 158n. 160; formulas of, 48; logical possibility of, 49; synthesizes law and will, 52
Categories: dynamical, 10; mathematical, 10

Causality: free, 14; intelligible, 11, 14, 15, 33, 34, 71; nontemporal, 12; rational, 27, 28, 31; of reason, 12; sensible, 11; synthetic character of, 9, 11; of the thing-in-itself, 11; unconditioned, 5, 18, 23
Cause: intelligible, 14, 15; spontaneity of, 6, 7
Character, 136n. 5; as an idea of reason, 34
Choice, 77–79, 82–87, 89–90, 92–94, 98, 100, 102, 111, 120, 123, 128n. 15, 151nn. 6, 22, 152nn. 31, 41, 153n. 50, 158n. 160
Christ, 159n. 19
Concepts: immanent use of, 22; rational, 23; sensible, 37; transcendent use of, 22
Conversion, 35, 110, 111
Cosmology, rational, 6
Credibilia, 68, 119
Critique of Practical Reason, xiii, xiv, 34, 46, 52, 54, 55, 56, 64, 65, 66, 68, 74, 83, 114, 119

Daval, Roger, 130n. 41
Delbos, Victor, xiii, xiv, 15, 34, 61, 119, 120, 150n. 1, 151n. 5, 155n. 102, 156n. 123
Deleuze, Gilles, 135n. 132, 158n. 160
Desire, faculty of, 84
Disposition, 95, 96, 98; inborn, 95
Duty, 26, 27, 46, 47, 49, 50, 56, 80, 81, 86, 91, 101, 105, 106, 114, 116, 117–21, 124, 135n. 4, 138n. 38, 150n. 18, 147n. 194, 151n. 16, 152n. 31, 158n. 160, 160n. 30; transcendental possibility of concept of, 50